CROCK POT COOKBOOK

FOR BEGINNERS 2024

1800 | Easy and Mouthwatering Recipes for Everyday Crock Pot Cooking to Live a Healthy Life

Lois T. Ellison

CONTENTS

Soups & Stews Recipes 38

Poultry Recipes 47

Beef, Pork & Lamb Recipes 56

Fish & Seafood Recipes 65

Lunch & Dinner Recipes 74

Side Dish Recipes 83

Snack Recipes | 92

Dessert Recipes | 100

Shopping List | 109

APPENDIX A: Measurement Conversions | 110

Appendix B : Recipes Index | 112

INTRODUCTION

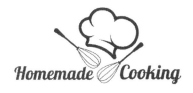

Homemade Cooking

Crafting this cookbook has been an extraordinary journey filled with love, passion, and the sheer joy of cooking. As an avid home cook, I've spent countless hours experimenting with the magical world of slow cooking, and it's been an adventure I couldn't wait to share with you.

The inspiration for this cookbook sprouted from my own experiences as a busy homemaker and a lover of hearty, homemade meals. In the heart of my cozy kitchen, my Crock Pot became my steadfast companion, transforming raw ingredients into flavorful masterpieces. With each recipe, I discovered the incredible convenience of setting and forgetting, allowing me to savor the precious moments spent with my family while a delicious dinner simmered away.

"The Crock Pot Cookbook" is the culmination of my lifelong love affair with slow cooking. Within these pages, you'll find a carefully curated collection of recipes that have graced my family's table for generations. From hearty stews to mouthwatering roasts and delectable desserts, each dish has been lovingly crafted, tested, and perfected to bring you the warmth and comfort of home-cooked meals.

But beyond the recipes, this cookbook is a reflection of who I am—an enthusiast of the simple yet profound pleasures of life. I'm a believer in the power of a home-cooked meal to bring people together, to create cherished memories, and to fill our hearts with contentment. I'm a firm advocate for the idea that anyone can embrace the art of slow cooking, regardless of their culinary background.

So, as you embark on this culinary journey with me, know that you are not only holding a cookbook but a piece of my heart and a taste of my cherished traditions. Together, let's discover the magic of the Crock Pot, relish the joy of preparing wholesome meals, and create lasting moments around the dinner table. Welcome to "The Crock Pot Cookbook" by Lois T. Ellison, where every recipe is an invitation to share in the simple pleasures of life.

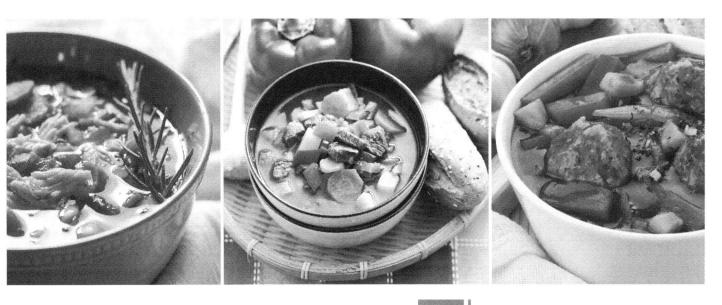

DEFINITION

A Crock Pot, also known as a slow cooker, is a versatile kitchen appliance designed for the methodical and gradual cooking of a wide array of dishes. This ingenious device operates on the principle of maintaining a low, steady heat over an extended period, allowing ingredients to meld and flavors to intensify while requiring minimal intervention from the cook. Crock Pots are renowned for their ability to turn simple, raw ingredients into tender, flavorful, and fully cooked meals, making them a valuable tool for home cooks seeking convenience and exceptional taste in their culinary creations.

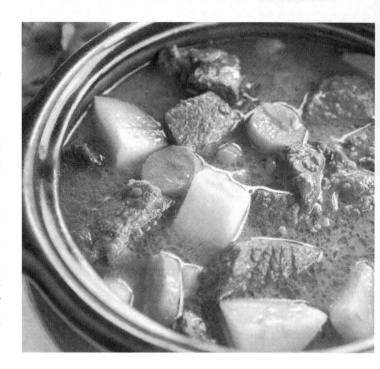

PARTS

Cooking Vessel: The heart of the Crock Pot is the cooking vessel, often made of durable ceramic or stoneware. This vessel is where the ingredients are placed and where the slow cooking magic happens.

Heating Element: Positioned beneath the cooking vessel, the heating element provides consistent and gentle heat to the contents, ensuring slow and even cooking.

Temperature Settings: Most Crock Pots feature multiple temperature settings, including "low," "high," and sometimes a "keep warm" setting. These settings empower users to adjust the cooking speed and temperature based on the recipe's requirements.

Lid: Crock Pots come equipped with a fitted lid, typically made of clear glass or durable plastic. The lid's primary function is to seal in heat and moisture, crucial for creating succulent and flavorful dishes.

Handles and Base: The housing of the Crock Pot often includes sturdy handles for safe and convenient transport. The base houses the control panel, including temperature settings and timers, in more modern models.

USERS

"Crock Pots are designed to cater to a wide range of individuals, making them a versatile kitchen appliance for various lifestyles and culinary needs. They are a boon for busy professionals and families, offering the convenience of preparing wholesome, homemade meals with minimal hands-on time. Furthermore, Crock Pots are suitable for home cooks of all skill levels, as they simplify meal preparation with clear instructions and minimal monitoring, building culinary confidence in beginners and offering experienced cooks the convenience and versatility of slow cooking. For those who prioritize healthy eating, slow cooking at lower temperatures in Crock Pots helps retain the nutrients in ingredients and allows for the use of lean cuts of meat and reduced fat.

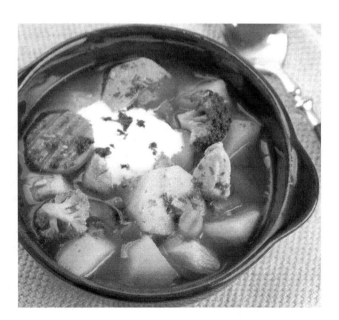

THE CANS AND CAN'TS OF USING A CROCK POT

cans

Preheat if Necessary

Some Crock Pot models require preheating before adding ingredients. Follow the manufacturer's recommendations for preheating, if applicable.

Layer Ingredients Thoughtfully

When preparing a recipe, layer ingredients thoughtfully. Place denser items, like root vegetables or meat, at the bottom to ensure even cooking. Delicate ingredients can be added on top.

Use Sufficient Liquid

Ensure there's enough liquid in your Crock Pot recipes to prevent them from drying out. Most slow cooker recipes require less liquid than traditional stovetop or oven cooking, but make sure to include at least some liquid.

Keep the Lid Closed

Avoid opening the lid frequently during cooking. Each time you open it, heat and moisture escape, which can significantly increase the cooking time.

Adjust Seasoning to Taste

Season your dishes conservatively at the beginning of cooking. You can always adjust the seasoning near the end of the cooking time to taste.

Plan Cooking Times

Plan your meals according to the recommended cooking times for specific recipes. Most Crock Pot recipes have suggested cooking durations for best results.

Thaw Ingredients

When using meat, poultry, or seafood, make sure they are thawed before adding them to the Crock Pot. This ensures even cooking and reduces the risk of foodborne illness.

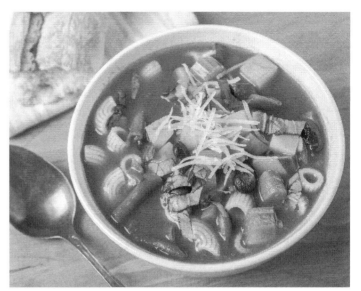

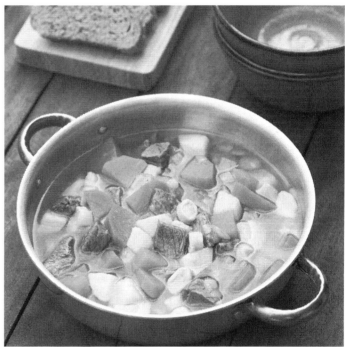

Use a Meat Thermometer

To ensure meat is thoroughly cooked, especially poultry and larger cuts, use a meat thermometer to check for safe internal temperatures.

can'ts

Can't Overfill

Avoid overfilling your Crock Pot. Most models should be filled between half to two-thirds full to ensure proper cooking and prevent spills.

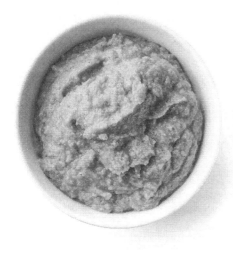 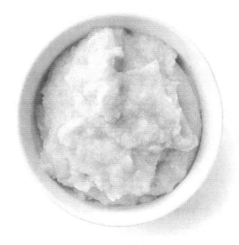 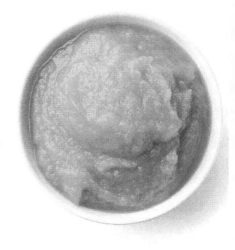

Can't Use Without Liquid

Never use a Crock Pot without any liquid. Adequate liquid is essential to prevent burning and sticking.

Can't Cook Frozen Ingredients

Do not add frozen ingredients directly to the Crock Pot. Thaw them first to ensure even cooking and food safety.

Can't Use Dairy Early

Dairy products (like milk or cream) can curdle if added too early in the cooking process. Add them toward the end of cooking.

Can't Cook Rice or Pasta for Too Long

Rice and pasta should be added later in the cooking process, as they can become mushy if cooked for the entire duration. Add them during the last hour or as specified in the recipe.

Can't Use Thin Cuts of Meat for Extended Cooking

Thin cuts of meat may become overly tender and fall apart during extended cooking. They are better suited for shorter cooking times.

Can't Store Leftovers in the Crock Pot

Avoid storing leftovers in the Crock Pot insert, as it may not cool down quickly enough, increasing the risk of bacterial growth. Transfer leftovers to separate containers and refrigerate promptly.

QUESTIONS YOU MAY HAVE ABOUT YOUR CROCK POT

● **How do I convert traditional recipes for use in a Crock Pot?**

Converting traditional recipes for a Crock Pot often involves adjusting cooking times and liquid quantities to suit the slow cooking method. Start by selecting recipes that are well-suited for slow cooking, such as stews, soups, or braised dishes. Generally, for every hour of conventional cooking, you'll need about 4-6 hours on the "low" setting or 1-2 hours on the "high" setting in a Crock Pot. Be mindful of overcooking, as slow cooking can intensify flavors. Additionally, consider the order in which ingredients are added, placing root vegetables and meats at the bottom for even cooking and tenderizing.

● **What size Crock Pot should I get for my family?**

Choosing the right Crock Pot size depends on your family size and meal requirements. A 3-4 quart Crock Pot is suitable for couples or small families, while a 6-8 quart model is better for larger households or for cooking larger cuts of meat. Consider your typical batch size and the types of meals you plan to prepare when selecting the appropriate size.

● **How do I prevent my Crock Pot meals from being too bland or too salty?**

Achieving the perfect flavor balance in Crock Pot meals requires an understanding of how flavors develop during slow cooking. Start by seasoning conservatively at the beginning and tasting as the dish progresses. Remember that flavors will intensify over time. To avoid oversalting, use low-sodium broth or seasonings initially and adjust near the end of cooking if needed. Adding fresh herbs and spices in the final hour can also enhance the overall taste.

● **Can I use my Crock Pot for making desserts and baked goods?**

Absolutely! Crock Pots are versatile enough to prepare a wide range of desserts, including puddings, cakes, cobblers, and even cheesecakes. Specialized dessert recipes are designed for slow cooking, taking advantage of the moist, gentle heat to create delicious treats. Follow dessert recipes specific to your Crock Pot for the best results.

● **How do I prevent food from sticking to the sides or burning at the bottom of the Crock Pot?**

Preventing sticking or burning requires thoughtful layering of ingredients. Place denser items, such as root vegetables or meat, at the bottom of the Crock Pot to ensure even cooking and to act as a buffer. Ensure there's enough liquid in the recipe, as adequate moisture helps prevent sticking. Some cooks also use cooking spray or slow cooker liners for added protection.

● **What do I do if my Crock Pot recipe turns out too thick or too thin?**

Adjusting the consistency of your dish is possible. If your dish turns out too thick, you can add additional

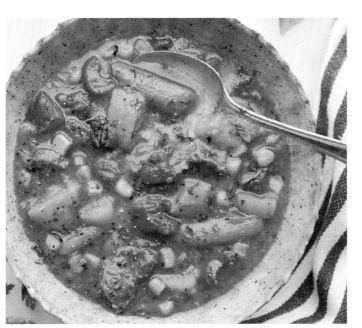

liquid, such as broth or water, to achieve the desired consistency. If it's too thin, you can create a slurry by mixing cornstarch or flour with a small amount of cold water, then gradually stir it into the Crock Pot. Allow it to simmer for a bit to thicken.

● **Are there any safety tips I should be aware of when using a Crock Pot?**

Ensuring safety while using a Crock Pot is essential. Place your Crock Pot on a stable, heat-resistant surface to prevent accidents. Avoid sudden temperature changes, such as placing a hot insert on a cold surface. Additionally, handle hot liquids with care and be cautious when opening the lid to prevent burns. For specific safety guidelines, consult your Crock Pot's user manual.

BEFORE YOU COOK

- Read the user manual.

- Select the right recipe.

- Gather and prepare ingredients.

- Preheat if required.

- Layer ingredients appropriately.

- Add enough liquid.

- Set temperature and timer.

- Secure the lid.

- Plug in the Crock Pot.

- Avoid frequent lid opening.

- Plan your schedule.

- Check for doneness.

- Adjust seasoning if necessary.

Crock Pot is a convenient and time-saving kitchen tool to help you reduce your busy time in the kitchen, and I hope you have fun cooking with the help of this Crock Pot Cookbook!

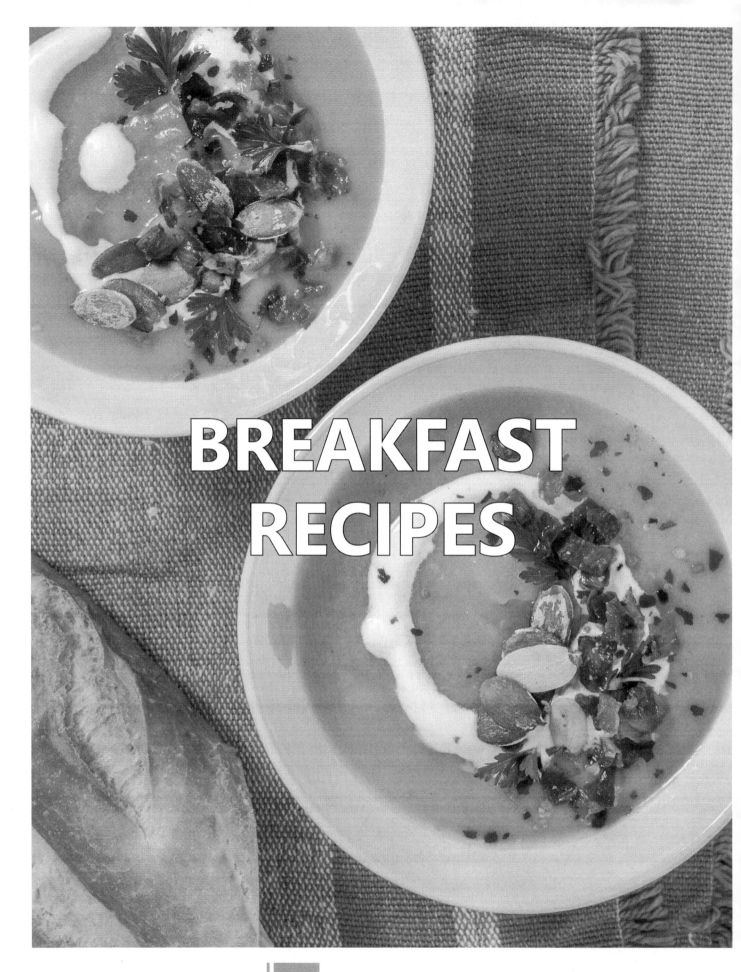

BREAKFAST RECIPES

Crock-pot Veggie Omelet

Servings: 4
Cooking Time: 2 Hours

Ingredients:
- 6 large eggs
- 4 cups spinach, fresh, chopped
- 1 ½ cups white mushrooms, sliced
- 2 cloves garlic, crushed
- 1 cup feta cheese, crumbled
- 2 tablespoons of coconut oil
- Salt and pepper to taste

Directions:
1. Heat the coconut oil in Crock-Pot. Set aside. In a mixing bowl, combine garlic, eggs, salt, and pepper. Add mushrooms and spinach to the mix. Cover and cook for about 2 hours, or until omelet is set. Check it at about 1 hour and 15 minutes into cooking time. When the omelet is cooked, add the feta and fold in half. Transfer to serving plate.

Nutrition Info:
- Calories: 659, Total Fat: 55.5 g, Saturated Fat: 30.3 g, Net Carbs: 7.7 g, Dietary Fiber: 2.8 g, Protein: 30.9 g

Tofu Eggs

Servings:4
Cooking Time: 7 Hours

Ingredients:
- 4 eggs, beaten
- 4 oz tofu, chopped
- ½ teaspoon curry paste
- 2 tablespoons coconut milk
- 1 teaspoon olive oil
- ½ teaspoon butter, melted

Directions:
1. Mix coconut milk with curry paste.
2. Then sprinkle the tofu with curry mixture.
3. After this, pour butter in the Crock Pot.
4. Add eggs, olive oil, and tofu mixture.

5. Close the lid and cook the meal on Low for 7 hours.

Nutrition Info:
- Per Serving: 118 calories, 8.1g protein, 1.4g carbohydrates, 9.4g fat, 0.4g fiber, 165mg cholesterol, 70mg sodium, 121mg potassium

Cowboy Breakfast Casserole

Servings:6
Cooking Time: 3 Hours

Ingredients:
- 1-pound ground beef
- 5 eggs, beaten
- 1 cup grass-fed Monterey Jack cheese, shredded
- Salt and pepper to taste
- 1 avocado, peeled and diced
- A handful of cilantro, chopped
- A dash of hot sauce

Directions:
1. In a skillet over medium flame, sauté the beef for three minutes until slightly golden.
2. Pour into the CrockPot and pour in eggs.
3. Sprinkle with cheese on top and season with salt and pepper to taste.
4. Close the lid and cook on high for 4 hours or on low for 6 hours.
5. Serve with avocado, cilantro and hot sauce.

Nutrition Info:
- Calories per serving: 439; Carbohydrates: 4.5g; Protein: 32.7g; Fat: 31.9g; Sugar: 0g; Sodium: 619mg; Fiber: 1.8g

Cheddar Eggs

Servings:4
Cooking Time: 2 Hours

Ingredients:
- 1 teaspoon butter, softened
- 4 eggs
- ½ teaspoon salt
- 1/3 cup Cheddar cheese, shredded

Directions:
1. Grease the Crock Pot bowl with butter and crack the eggs inside.
2. Sprinkle the eggs with salt and shredded cheese.
3. Close the lid and cook on High for 2 hours.

Nutrition Info:
- Per Serving: 109 calories, 7.9g protein, 0.5g carbohydrates, 8.5g fat, 0g fiber, 176mg cholesterol, 418mg sodium, 69mg potassium.

Corn Casserole

Servings:6
Cooking Time: 8 Hours

Ingredients:
- 1 cup sweet corn kernels
- 1 chili pepper, chopped
- 1 tomato, chopped
- 1 cup Mozzarella, shredded
- 2 tablespoons cream cheese
- 5 oz ham, chopped
- 1 teaspoon garlic powder
- 2 eggs, beaten

Directions:
1. Mix sweet corn kernels, with chili pepper, tomato, and ham.
2. Add minced garlic and stir the ingredients.
3. Transfer it in the Crock Pot and flatten gently.
4. Top the casserole with eggs, cream cheese, and Mozzarella.
5. Cook the casserole on LOW for 8 hours.

Nutrition Info:
- Per Serving: 110 calories, 8.3g protein, 7.2g carbohydrates, 5.8g fat, 1g fiber, 74mg cholesterol, 449mg sodium, 159mg potassium.

Breakfast Monkey Bread

Servings:6
Cooking Time: 6 Hours

Ingredients:
- 10 oz biscuit rolls
- 1 tablespoon ground cardamom
- 1 tablespoon sugar
- 2 tablespoons coconut oil
- 1 egg, beaten

Directions:
1. Chop the biscuit roll roughly.
2. Mix sugar with ground cardamom.
3. Melt the coconut oil.
4. Put the ½ part of chopped biscuit rolls in the Crock Pot in one layer and sprinkle with melted coconut oil and ½ part of all ground cinnamon mixture.
5. Then top it with remaining biscuit roll chops and sprinkle with cardamom mixture and coconut oil.
6. Then brush the bread with a beaten egg and close the lid.
7. Cook the meal on High for 6 hours.
8. Cook the cooked bread well.

Nutrition Info:
- Per Serving: 178 calories, 6.1g protein, 26.4g carbohydrates, 7g fat, 2g fiber, 27mg cholesterol, 238mg sodium, 21mg potassium.

Cauliflower Rice Pudding

Servings: 2
Cooking Time: 2 Hours

Ingredients:
- ¼ cup maple syrup
- 3 cups almond milk
- 1 cup cauliflower rice
- 2 tablespoons vanilla extract

Directions:
1. Put cauliflower rice in your Crock Pot, add maple syrup, almond milk and vanilla extract, stir, cover and cook on High for 2 hours.
2. Stir your pudding again, divide into bowls and serve for breakfast.

Nutrition Info:
- calories 240, fat 2, fiber 2, carbs 15, protein 5

Hot Eggs Mix

Servings: 2
Cooking Time: 2 Hours

Ingredients:
- Cooking spray
- 4 eggs, whisked
- ¼ cup sour cream
- A pinch of salt and black pepper
- ½ teaspoon chili powder
- ½ teaspoon hot paprika
- ½ red bell pepper, chopped
- ½ yellow onion, chopped
- 2 cherry tomatoes, cubed
- 1 tablespoon parsley, chopped

Directions:
1. In a bowl, mix the eggs with the cream, salt, pepper and the other ingredients except the cooking spray and whisk well.
2. Grease your Crock Pot with cooking spray, pour the eggs mix inside, spread, stir, put the lid on and cook on High for 2 hours.
3. Divide the mix between plates and serve.

Nutrition Info:
- calories 162, fat 5, fiber 7, carbs 15, protein 4

Veggie Omelet

Servings: 4
Cooking Time: 2 Hours

Ingredients:
- ½ cup milk
- 6 eggs
- Salt and black pepper to the taste
- A pinch of chili powder
- A pinch of garlic powder
- 1 red bell pepper, chopped
- 1 cup broccoli florets
- 1 yellow onion, chopped
- 1 garlic clove, minced
- 1 tablespoon cheddar cheese, shredded
- Cooking spray

Directions:
1. In a bowl, mix the eggs with milk, salt, pepper, chili powder, garlic powder, broccoli, garlic, bell pepper and onion and whisk well.
2. Grease your Crock Pot with cooking spray, add eggs mix, spread, cover Crock Pot and cook on High

for 2 hours.
3. Slice omelet, divide it between plates and serve hot for breakfast.

Nutrition Info:
- calories 142, fat 7, fiber 1, carbs 8, protein 10

Pumpkin And Berries Bowls

Servings: 2
Cooking Time: 4 Hours

Ingredients:
- ½ cup coconut cream
- 1 and ½ cups pumpkin, peeled and cubed
- 1 cup blackberries
- 2 tablespoons maple syrup
- ¼ teaspoon nutmeg, ground
- ½ teaspoon vanilla extract

Directions:
1. In your Crock Pot, combine the pumpkin with the berries, cream and the other ingredients, toss, put the lid on and cook on Low for 4 hours.
2. Divide into bowls and serve for breakfast!

Nutrition Info:
- calories 120, fat 2, fiber 2, carbs 4, protein 2

Almond And Quinoa Bowls

Servings: 2
Cooking Time: 5 Hours

Ingredients:
- 1 cup quinoa
- 2 cups almond milk
- 2 tablespoons butter, melted
- 2 tablespoons brown sugar
- A pinch of cinnamon powder
- A pinch of nutmeg, ground
- ¼ cup almonds, sliced
- Cooking spray

Directions:
1. Grease your Crock Pot with the cooking spray, add the quinoa, milk, melted butter and the other ingredients, toss, put the lid on and cook on Low for 5 hours.
2. Divide the mix into bowls and serve for breakfast.

Nutrition Info:
- calories 211, fat 3, fiber 6, carbs 12, protein 5

Hash Browns And Sausage Casserole

Servings: 12
Cooking Time: 4 Hours

Ingredients:
- 30 ounces hash browns
- 1 pound sausage, browned and sliced
- 8 ounces mozzarella cheese, shredded
- 8 ounces cheddar cheese, shredded
- 6 green onions, chopped
- ½ cup milk
- 12 eggs
- Cooking spray
- Salt and black pepper to the taste

Directions:
1. Grease your Crock Pot with cooking spray and add half of the hash browns, half of the sausage, half of the mozzarella, cheddar and green onions.
2. In a bowl, mix the eggs with salt, pepper and milk and whisk well.
3. Add half of the eggs mix into the Crock Pot, then layer the remaining hash browns, sausages, mozzarella, cheddar and green onions.
4. Top with the rest of the eggs, cover the Crock Pot and cook on High for 4 hours.
5. Divide between plates and serve hot.

Nutrition Info:
- calories 300, fat 3, fiber 7, carbs 10, protein 12

Baguette Boats

Servings:4
Cooking Time: 3 Hours

Ingredients:
- 6 oz baguette (2 baguettes)
- 4 ham slices
- 1 teaspoon minced garlic
- ½ cup Mozzarella, shredded
- 1 teaspoon olive oil
- 1 egg, beaten

Directions:
1. Cut the baguettes into the halves and remove the flesh from the bread.
2. Chop the ham and mix it with egg, Mozzarella, and minced garlic.
3. Fill the baguettes with ham mixture.
4. Then brush the Crock Pot bowl with olive oil from inside.

5. Put the baguette boats in the Crock Pot and close the lid.
6. Cook them for 3 hours on High.

Nutrition Info:
- Per Serving: 205 calories, 12.1g protein, 25.5g carbohydrates, 6.1g fat, 1.4g fiber, 59mg cholesterol, 678mg sodium, 152mg potassium.

Creamy Bacon Millet

Servings: 6
Cooking Time: 4 Hrs 10 Minutes

Ingredients:
- 3 cup millet
- 6 cup chicken stock
- 1 tsp salt
- 4 tbsp heavy cream
- 5 oz. bacon, chopped

Directions:
1. Add millet and chicken stock to the Crock Pot.
2. Stir in chopped bacon and salt.
3. Put the cooker's lid on and set the cooking time to 4 hours on High settings.
4. Stir in cream and again cover the lid of the Crock Pot.
5. Cook for 10 minutes on High setting.
6. Serve.

Nutrition Info:
- Per Serving: Calories 572, Total Fat 17.8g, Fiber 9g, Total Carbs 83.09g, Protein 20g

Creamy Asparagus Chicken

Servings: 7
Cooking Time: 8 Hrs

Ingredients:
- 1 cup cream
- 2 lb. chicken breast, skinned, boneless, sliced
- 1 tsp chili powder
- 3 tbsp flour
- 1 tsp oregano
- 1 tsp ground white pepper
- 1 tsp sriracha
- 6 oz. asparagus
- 1 tsp sage

Directions:
1. Whisk chili powder, oregano, sage, white pepper, and flour in a shallow tray.

2. Add the chicken slices to this spice mixture and coat them well.

3. Now add cream, chopped veggies, and Sriracha to the Crock Pot.

4. Place the coated chicken slices in the cooker.

5. Put the cooker's lid on and set the cooking time to 8 hours on Low settings.

6. Serve warm.

Nutrition Info:

• Per Serving: Calories 311, Total Fat 18.8g, Fiber 1g, Total Carbs 5.71g, Protein 29g

Vanilla Yogurt

Servings: 8
Cooking Time: 10 Hrs

Ingredients:

• 3 tsp gelatin
• ½ gallon milk
• 7 oz. plain yogurt
• 1 and ½ tbsp vanilla extract
• ½ cup maple syrup

Directions:

1. Add milk to the Crock Pot to heat it up.

2. Put the cooker's lid on and set the cooking time to 3 hours on Low settings.

3. Take 1 cup of this hot milk in a bowl and stir in gelatin.

4. Now take another cup of milk in another bowl and add yogurt.

5. Mix well, then pour into the Crock Pot.

6. Add the gelatin-milk mixture, maple syrup, and vanilla.

7. Put the cooker's lid on and set the cooking time to 7 hours on Low settings.

8. Allow it to cool then serve.

Nutrition Info:

• Per Serving: Calories 200, Total Fat 4g, Fiber 5g, Total Carbs 10g, Protein 5g

Breakfast Lasagna

Servings:10
Cooking Time: 4-5 Hours

Ingredients:

• 1 small onion, diced
• 10 ounces lean ground beef
• 2 garlic cloves, minced

• 2 tablespoons olive oil
• ½ teaspoon sea salt
• 6 large eggs
• 1 cup ricotta cheese
• 1 cup mozzarella cheese, grated
• 1 cup feta cheese
• 2 cups spinach, fresh chopped
• 2 medium eggplants, cut into ½-inch slices
• 1 large zucchini, cut into ½-inch slices
• 1 cup marinara sauce, no-sugar-added

Nutrition Info:

• Calories: 537, Total Fat: 46 g, Saturated Fat: 19.6 g, Net Carbs: 11.4 g, Dietary Fiber: 5.4 g, Protein: 33 g

Turkey Breakfast Casserole

Servings: 8
Cooking Time: 8 Hours 30 Minutes

Ingredients:

• 1-pound turkey sausages, cooked and drained
• 1 dozen eggs
• 1 (30 oz) package shredded hash browns, thawed
• 1 yellow onion, chopped
• 2 cups Colby Jack cheese, shredded
• 1 cup milk
• 1 teaspoon salt
• ½ teaspoon red pepper flakes, crushed
• 4 tablespoons flour
• ½ teaspoon black pepper

Directions:

1. Grease a crockpot and layer with 1/3 of the hash browns, onions, sausages and cheese.

2. Repeat these layers twice ending with the layer of cheese.

3. Whisk together the rest of the ingredients in a large mixing bowl.

4. Transfer this mixture into the crockpot and cover the lid.

5. Cover and cook on LOW for about 8 hours.

6. Dish out to serve the delicious breakfast.

Nutrition Info:

• Calories: 453 Fat: 25g Carbohydrates: 26g

Potato And Ham Mix

Servings: 2
Cooking Time: 6 Hours

Ingredients:
- Cooking spray
- 4 eggs, whisked
- ½ cup red potatoes, peeled and grated
- ¼ cup heavy cream
- ¼ cup ham, chopped
- 1 tablespoon cilantro, chopped
- ½ teaspoon turmeric powder
- Salt and black pepper to the taste

Directions:
1. Grease your Crock Pot with cooking spray, add the eggs, potatoes and the other ingredients, whisk, put the lid on and cook on High for 6 hours.
2. Divide between plates and serve for breakfast.

Nutrition Info:
- calories 200, fat 4, fiber 6, carbs 12, protein 6

Quinoa And Oats Mix

Servings: 6
Cooking Time: 7 Hours

Ingredients:
- ½ cup quinoa
- 1 and ½ cups steel cut oats
- 4 and ½ cups almond milk
- 2 tablespoons maple syrup
- 4 tablespoons brown sugar
- 1 and ½ teaspoons vanilla extract
- Cooking spray

Directions:
1. Grease your Crock Pot with cooking spray, add quinoa, oats, almond milk, maple syrup, sugar and vanilla extract, cover and cook on Low for 7 hours.
2. Stir, divide into bowls and serve for breakfast.

Nutrition Info:
- calories 251, fat 8, fiber 8, carbs 20, protein 5

Carrots Oatmeal

Servings: 2
Cooking Time: 8 Hours

Ingredients:
- ½ cup old fashioned oats
- 1 cup almond milk
- 2 carrots, peeled and grated
- ½ teaspoon cinnamon powder
- 2 tablespoons brown sugar
- ¼ cup walnuts, chopped
- Cooking spray

Directions:
1. Grease your Crock Pot with cooking spray, add the oats, milk, carrots and the other ingredients, toss, put the lid on and cook on Low for 8 hours.
2. Divide the oatmeal into 2 bowls and serve.

Nutrition Info:
- calories 590, fat 40.7, fiber 9.1, carbs 49.9, protein 12

Feta And Eggs Muffins

Servings:2
Cooking Time: 6 Hours

Ingredients:
- 2 eggs, beaten
- 2 teaspoons cream cheese
- 1 oz feta, crumbled
- 1 oz fresh cilantro, chopped
- ½ teaspoon chili powder
- 1 teaspoon butter, melted

Directions:
1. Mix all ingredients and pour in the silicone muffin molds.
2. After this, transfer the muffin molds in the Crock Pot.
3. Cook the breakfast on Low for 6 hours.

Nutrition Info:
- Per Serving: 134 calories, 8.2g protein, 1.9g carbohydrates, 10.6g fat, 0.6g fiber, 185mg cholesterol, 256mg sodium, 159mg potassium

Herbed Pork Meatballs

Servings: 9
Cooking Time: 4 Hrs

Ingredients:
- 2 lb. ground pork
- 1 tbsp dried parsley
- 1 tsp dried dill
- 1 tsp paprika
- 1 tsp salt
- 1 egg
- 1 tbsp semolina
- ½ cup tomato juice
- 3 tbsp flour
- 1 tbsp minced garlic
- 1 tsp onion powder
- 1 tsp sugar
- 1 tsp chives
- 1 oz. bay leaves

Directions:
1. Beat egg in a bowl then stir in ground pork, parsley, dill, salt, paprika, garlic, semolina, and onion powder in a large bowl.
2. Make medium-sized meatballs out of this mixture.
3. Cover the base of your Crock Pot with a parchment sheet.
4. Place the meatballs in the cooker.
5. Now mix tomato juice, flour, bay leaf, sugar and chives in a separate bowl.
6. Pour this mixture over the meatballs.
7. Put the cooker's lid on and set the cooking time to 4 hours on Low settings.
8. Serve the meatballs with their sauce.

Nutrition Info:
- Per Serving: Calories 344, Total Fat 22.4g, Fiber 1g, Total Carbs 6.87g, Protein 28g

Romano Cheese Frittata

Servings:4
Cooking Time: 3 Hours

Ingredients:
- 4 oz Romano cheese, grated
- 5 eggs, beaten
- ¼ cup of coconut milk
- ½ cup bell pepper, chopped
- ½ teaspoon ground white pepper
- 1 teaspoon olive oil
- ½ teaspoon ground coriander

Directions:
1. Mix eggs with coconut milk, ground white pepper, bell pepper, and ground coriander.
2. Then brush the Crock Pot bowl with olive oil.
3. Pour the egg mixture in the Crock Pot.
4. Cook the frittata on High for 2.5 hours.
5. Then top the frittata with Romano cheese and cook for 30 minutes on High.

Nutrition Info:
- Per Serving: 238 calories, 16.5g protein, 3.6g carbohydrates, 17.9g fat, 0.6g fiber, 234mg cholesterol, 420mg sodium, 169mg potassium.

Cranberry Almond Quinoa

Servings: 4
Cooking Time: 2 Hrs

Ingredients:
- 3 cups of coconut water
- 1 tsp vanilla extract
- 1 cup quinoa
- 3 tsp honey
- 1/8 cup almonds, sliced
- 1/8 cup coconut flakes
- ¼ cup cranberries, dried

Directions:
1. Add coconut water, honey, vanilla, quinoa, almonds, cranberries, and coconut flakes to the Crock Pot.
2. Put the cooker's lid on and set the cooking time to 2 hours on High settings.
3. Dish out and serve.

Nutrition Info:
- Per Serving: Calories 261, Total Fat 7g, Fiber 8g, Total Carbs 18g, Protein 4g

Sweet Eggs

Servings:4
Cooking Time: 4 Hours

Ingredients:
- 4 oz white bread, chopped
- 2 tablespoons sugar
- 6 eggs, beaten
- ¼ cup milk
- 1 teaspoon vanilla extract
- 1 teaspoon avocado oil

Directions:
1. Mix eggs with sugar and milk. Add vanilla extract and bread.
2. Then brush the Crock Pot bottom with avocado oil.
3. Pour the egg mixture inside and close the lid.
4. Cook the meal on Low for 4 hours.

Nutrition Info:
- Per Serving: 204 calories, 11g protein, 21.8g carbohydrates, 8g fat, 0.7g fiber, 247mg cholesterol, 293mg sodium, 131mg potassium

Turkey Omelet

Servings:4
Cooking Time: 5 Hours

Ingredients:
- ½ teaspoon garlic powder
- 6 oz ground turkey
- 4 eggs, beaten
- 1 tablespoon coconut oil
- ½ teaspoon salt
- ¼ cup milk

Directions:
1. Mix milk with salt, eggs, and garlic powder. Then add ground turkey.
2. Grease the Crock Pot bowl bottom with coconut oil.
3. Put the egg mixture in the Crock Pot, flatten it, and close the lid.
4. Cook the omelet on Low for 5 hours.

Nutrition Info:
- Per Serving: 184 calories, 17.7g protein, 1.3g carbohydrates, 12.8g fat, 0g fiber, 208mg cholesterol, 405mg sodium, 186mg potassium

Peach Oats

Servings:3
Cooking Time: 7 Hours

Ingredients:
- ½ cup steel cut oats
- 1 cup milk
- ½ cup peaches, pitted, chopped
- 1 teaspoon ground cardamom

Directions:
1. Mix steel-cut oats with milk and pour the mixture in the Crock Pot.
2. Add ground cardamom and peaches. Stir the ingredients gently and close the lid.
3. Cook the meal on low for 7 hours.

Nutrition Info:
- Per Serving: 159 calories, 7g protein, 24.8g carbohydrates, 3.8g fat, 3.2g fiber, 7mg cholesterol, 38mg sodium, 200mg potassium

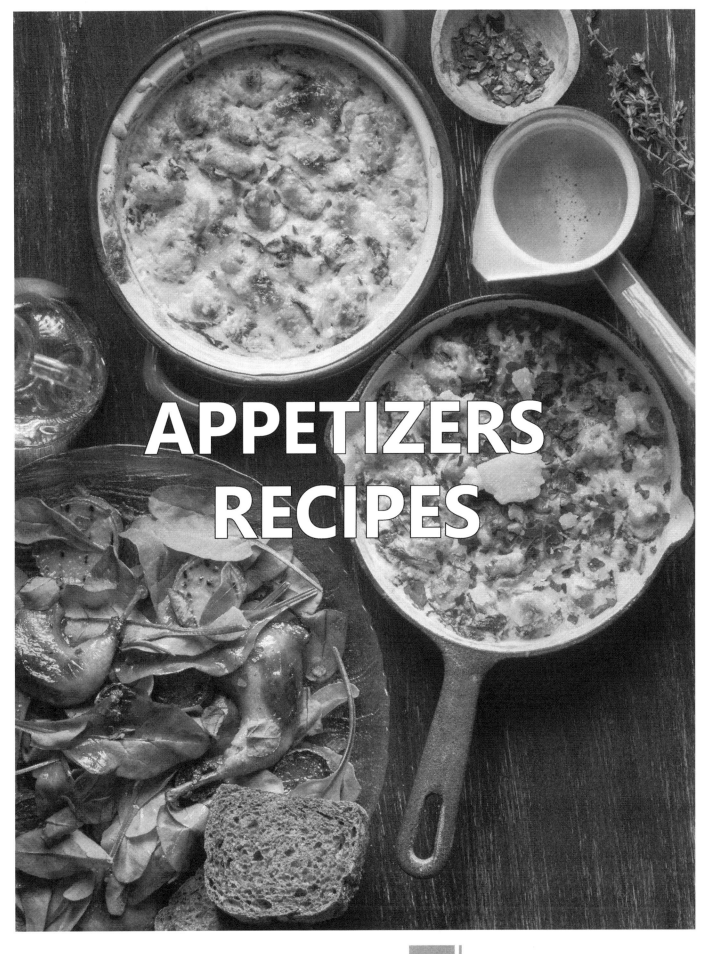

APPETIZERS RECIPES

Hoisin Chicken Wings

Servings: 8
Cooking Time: 7 1/4 Hours

Ingredients:
- 4 pounds chicken wings
- 2/3 cup hoisin sauce
- 4 garlic cloves, minced
- 1 teaspoon grated ginger
- 1 teaspoon sesame oil
- 1 tablespoon molasses
- 1 teaspoon hot sauce
- 1/4 teaspoon ground black pepper
- 1/2 teaspoon salt

Directions:
1. Mix the hoisin sauce, garlic, ginger, sesame oil, molasses, hot sauce, black pepper and salt in your Crock Pot.
2. Add the chicken wings and toss them around until evenly coated.
3. Cover with a lid and cook on low settings for 7 hours.
4. Serve the wings warm or chilled.

Queso Verde Dip

Servings: 12
Cooking Time: 4 1/4 Hours

Ingredients:
- 1 pound ground chicken
- 2 shallots, chopped
- 2 tablespoons olive oil
- 2 cups salsa verde
- 1 cup cream cheese
- 2 cups grated Cheddar
- 2 poblano peppers, chopped
- 1 tablespoon Worcestershire sauce
- 4 garlic cloves, minced
- 1/4 cup chopped cilantro
- Salt and pepper to taste

Directions:
1. Combine all the ingredients in your Crock Pot.

2. Add salt and pepper to taste and cook on low heat for 4 hours.
3. The dip is best served warm.

Turkey Meatloaf

Servings: 8
Cooking Time: 6 1/4 Hours

Ingredients:
- 1 1/2 pounds ground turkey
- 1 carrot, grated
- 1 sweet potato, grated
- 1 egg
- 1/4 cup breadcrumbs
- 1/4 teaspoon chili powder
- Salt and pepper to taste
- 1 cup shredded mozzarella

Directions:
1. Mix all the ingredients in a bowl and season with salt and pepper as needed.
2. Give it a good mix then transfer the mixture in your Crock Pot.
3. Level the mixture well and cover with the pot's lid.
4. Cook on low settings for 6 hours.
5. Serve the meatloaf warm or chilled.

Roasted Bell Peppers Dip

Servings: 8
Cooking Time: 2 1/4 Hours

Ingredients:
- 4 roasted red bell peppers, drained
- 2 cans chickpeas, drained
- 1/2 cup water
- 1 shallot, chopped
- 4 garlic cloves, minced
- Salt and pepper to taste
- 2 tablespoons lemon juice
- 2 tablespoons olive oil

Directions:
1. Combine the bell peppers, chickpeas, water, shallot and garlic in a Crock Pot.

2. Add salt and pepper as needed and cook on high settings for 2 hours.

3. When done, puree the dip in a blender, adding the lemon juice and olive oil as well.

4. Serve the dip fresh or store it in the fridge in an air-tight container for up to 2 days.

Bean Queso

Servings: 10
Cooking Time: 6 1/4 Hours

Ingredients:
- 1 can black beans, drained
- 1 cup chopped green chiles
- 1/2 cup red salsa
- 1 teaspoon dried oregano
- 1/2 teaspoon cumin powder
- 1 cup light beer
- 1 1/2 cups grated Cheddar
- Salt and pepper to taste

Directions:
1. Combine the beans, chiles, oregano, cumin, salsa, beer and cheese in your Crock Pot.

2. Add salt and pepper as needed and cook on low settings for 6 hours.

3. Serve the bean queso warm.

Beer Cheese Fondue

Servings: 8
Cooking Time: 2 1/4 Hours

Ingredients:
- 1 shallot, chopped
- 1 garlic clove, minced
- 1 cup grated Gruyere cheese
- 2 cups grated Cheddar
- 1 tablespoon cornstarch
- 1 teaspoon Dijon mustard
- 1/2 teaspoon cumin seeds
- 1 cup beer
- Salt and pepper to taste

Directions:
1. Combine the shallot, garlic, cheeses, cornstarch, mustard, cumin seeds and beer in your Crock Pot.

2. Add salt and pepper to taste and mix well.

3. Cover the pot with its lid and cook on high settings for 2 hours.

4. Serve the fondue warm.

Mexican Chili Dip

Servings: 20
Cooking Time: 2 1/4 Hours

Ingredients:
- 1 can black beans, drained
- 1 can red beans, drained
- 1 can diced tomatoes
- 1/2 teaspoon cumin powder
- 1/2 teaspoon chili powder
- 1/2 cup beef stock
- Salt and pepper to taste
- 1 1/2 cups grated Cheddar

Directions:
1. Combine the beans, tomatoes, cumin powder, chili and stock in your Crock Pot.

2. Add salt and pepper to taste and top with grated cheese.

3. Cook on high settings for 2 hours.

4. The dip is best served warm.

Artichoke Bread Pudding

Servings: 10
Cooking Time: 6 1/2 Hours

Ingredients:
- 6 cups bread cubes
- 6 artichoke hearts, drained and chopped
- 1/2 cup grated Parmesan
- 4 eggs
- 1/2 cup sour cream
- 1 cup milk
- 4 oz. spinach, chopped
- 1 tablespoon chopped parsley
- 2 tablespoons olive oil
- Salt and pepper to taste
- 1/2 teaspoon dried oregano
- 1/2 teaspoon dried basil

Directions:
1. Combine the bread cubes, artichoke hearts and Parmesan in your Crock Pot. Add the spinach and parsley as well.

2. In a bowl, mix the eggs, sour cream, milk, oregano and basil, as well as salt and pepper.

3. Pour this mixture over the bread and press the bread slightly to make sure it soaks up all the liquid.

4. Cover the pot with its lid and cook on low settings for 6 hours.

5. The bread can be served both warm and chilled.

Mozzarella Stuffed Meatballs

Servings: 8
Cooking Time: 6 1/2 Hours

Ingredients:
- 2 pounds ground chicken
- 1 teaspoon dried basil
- 1/2 teaspoon dried oregano
- 1 egg
- 1/2 cup breadcrumbs
- Salt and pepper to taste
- Mini-mozzarella balls as needed
- 1/2 cup chicken stock

Directions:
1. Mix the ground chicken, basil, oregano, egg, breadcrumbs, salt and pepper in a bowl.
2. Take small pieces of the meat mixture and flatten it in your palm. Place a mozzarella ball in the center and gather the meat around the mozzarella.
3. Shape the meatballs, making sure they are well sealed and place them in a Crock Pot.
4. Add the chicken stock and cook on low settings for 6 hours.
5. Serve the meatballs warm or chilled.

Spanish Chorizo Dip

Servings: 8
Cooking Time: 6 1/4 Hours

Ingredients:
- 8 chorizo links, diced
- 1 can diced tomatoes
- 1 chili pepper, chopped
- 1 cup cream cheese
- 2 cups grated Cheddar cheese
- 1/4 cup white wine

Directions:
1. Combine all the ingredients in your Crock Pot.
2. Cook the dip on low settings for 6 hours.
3. Serve the dip warm.

Pimiento Cheese Dip

Servings: 8
Cooking Time: 2 1/4 Hours

Ingredients:
- 1/2 pound grated Cheddar
- 1/4 pound grated pepper Jack cheese
- 1/2 cup sour cream
- 1/2 cup green olives, sliced
- 2 tablespoons diced pimientos
- 1 teaspoon hot sauce
- 1/4 teaspoon garlic powder
- 1/4 teaspoon onion powder

Directions:
1. Combine all the ingredients in a Crock Pot.
2. Cover the pot with its lid and cook on high settings for 2 hours.
3. The dip is best served warm with vegetable sticks or bread sticks.

Pretzel Party Mix

Servings: 10
Cooking Time: 2 1/4 Hours

Ingredients:
- 4 cups pretzels
- 1 cup peanuts
- 1 cup pecans
- 1 cup crispy rice cereals
- 1/4 cup butter, melted
- 1 teaspoon Worcestershire sauce
- 1 teaspoon salt
- 1 teaspoon garlic powder

Directions:
1. Combine the pretzels, peanuts, pecans and rice cereals in your Crock Pot.
2. Drizzle with melted butter and Worcestershire sauce and mix well then sprinkle with salt and garlic powder.
3. Cover and cook on high settings for 2 hours, mixing once during cooking.
4. Allow to cool before serving.

Beer Bbq Meatballs

Servings: 10
Cooking Time: 7 1/2 Hours

Ingredients:
- 2 pounds ground pork
- 1 pound ground beef
- 1 carrot, grated
- 2 shallots, chopped
- 1 egg
- 1/2 cup breadcrumbs
- 1/2 teaspoon cumin powder
- Salt and pepper to taste
- 1 cup dark beer
- 1 cup BBQ sauce
- 1 bay leaf
- 1/2 teaspoon chili powder
- 1 teaspoon apple cider vinegar

Directions:
1. Mix the ground pork and beef in a bowl. Add the carrot, shallots, egg, breadcrumbs, cumin, salt and pepper and mix well. Form small meatballs and place them on your chopping board.
2. For the beer sauce, combine the beer, BBQ sauce, bay leaf, chili powder and vinegar in a Crock Pot.
3. Place the meatballs in the pot and cover with its lid.
4. Cook on low settings for 7 hours.
5. Serve the meatballs warm or chilled.

Nacho Sauce

Servings: 12
Cooking Time: 6 1/4 Hours

Ingredients:
- 2 pounds ground beef
- 2 tablespoons Mexican seasoning
- 1 teaspoon chili powder
- 1 can diced tomatoes
- 2 shallots, chopped
- 4 garlic cloves, minced
- 1 can sweet corn, drained
- 2 cups grated Cheddar cheese

Directions:
1. Combine all the ingredients in your Crock Pot.
2. Cook on low settings for 6 hours.
3. This dip is best served warm.

Spicy Chicken Taquitos

Servings: 8
Cooking Time: 6 1/2 Hours

Ingredients:
- 4 chicken breasts, cooked and diced
- 1 cup cream cheese
- 2 jalapeno peppers, chopped
- 1/2 cup canned sweet corn, drained
- 1/2 teaspoon cumin powder
- 4 garlic cloves, minced
- 16 taco-sized flour tortillas
- 2 cups grated Cheddar cheese

Directions:
1. In a bowl, mix the chicken, cream cheese, garlic, cumin, poblano peppers and corn. Stir in the cheese as well.
2. Place your tortillas on your working surface and top each tortilla with the cheese mixture.
3. Roll the tortillas tightly to form an even roll.
4. Place the rolls in your Crock Pot.
5. Cook on low settings for 6 hours.
6. Serve warm.

Ranch Turkey Bites

Servings: 6
Cooking Time: 7 1/4 Hours

Ingredients:
- 2 pounds turkey breast, cubed
- 1 carrot, sliced
- 1/2 teaspoon garlic powder
- 1 tablespoon Ranch dressing seasoning
- 1 teaspoon hot sauce
- 1 cup tomato sauce
- Salt and pepper to taste

Directions:
1. Combine all the ingredients in a Crock Pot.
2. Mix well until the ingredients are well distributed and adjust the taste with salt and pepper.
3. Cover with a lid and cook on low settings for 7 hours.
4. Serve the turkey bites warm or chilled.

Creamy Potatoes

Servings: 6
Cooking Time: 6 1/4 Hours

Ingredients:

- 3 pounds small new potatoes, washed
- 4 bacon slices, chopped
- 1 teaspoon dried oregano
- 1 shallot, chopped
- 2 tablespoons olive oil
- 2 garlic cloves, chopped
- Salt and pepper to taste
- 1 cup sour cream
- 2 green onions, chopped
- 2 tablespoons chopped parsley

Directions:

1. Combine the potatoes, bacon, oregano, shallot, olive oil and garlic in a Crock Pot.
2. Add salt and pepper and mix until the ingredients are well distributed.
3. Cover the pot with its lid and cook on low settings for 6 hours.
4. When done, mix the cooked potatoes with sour cream, onions and parsley and serve right away.

Eggplant Caviar

Servings: 6
Cooking Time: 3 1/4 Hours

Ingredients:

- 2 large eggplants, peeled and cubed
- 4 tablespoons olive oil
- 1 teaspoon dried basil
- 1 teaspoon dried oregano
- 1 lemon, juiced
- 2 garlic cloves, minced
- Salt and pepper to taste

Directions:

1. Combine the eggplant cubes, olive oil, basil and oregano in a Crock Pot.
2. Add salt and pepper to taste and cook on high settings for 3 hours.
3. When done, stir in the lemon juice, garlic, salt and pepper and mash the mix well with a potato masher.
4. Serve the dip chilled.

Bacon Wrapped Dates

Servings: 8
Cooking Time: 1 3/4 Hours

Ingredients:

- 16 dates, pitted
- 16 almonds
- 16 slices bacon

Directions:

1. Stuff each date with an almond.
2. Wrap each date in bacon and place the wrapped dates in your Crock Pot.
3. Cover with its lid and cook on high settings for 1 1/4 hours.
4. Serve warm or chilled.

Sweet Corn Jalapeno Dip

Servings: 10
Cooking Time: 2 1/4 Hours

Ingredients:

- 4 bacon slices, chopped
- 3 cans sweet corn, drained
- 4 jalapenos, seeded and chopped
- 1 cup sour cream
- 1 cup grated Cheddar cheese
- 1/2 cup cream cheese
- 1 pinch nutmeg
- 2 tablespoons chopped cilantro

Directions:

1. Combine the corn, jalapenos, sour cream, Cheddar, cream cheese and nutmeg in a Crock Pot.
2. Cook on high settings for 2 hours.
3. When done, stir in the cilantro and serve the dip warm.
4. Store it in an airtight container in the fridge for up to 2 days. Re-heat it when need it.

Cranberry Baked Brie

Servings: 6
Cooking Time: 2 1/4 Hours

Ingredients:
- 1 wheel of Brie
- 1/2 cup cranberry sauce
- 1/2 teaspoon dried thyme

Directions:
1. Spoon the cranberry sauce in your Crock Pot.
2. Sprinkle with thyme and top with the Brie cheese.
3. Cover with a lid and cook on low settings for 2 hours.
4. The cheese is best served warm with bread sticks or tortilla chips.

Stuffed Artichokes

Servings: 6
Cooking Time: 6 1/2 Hours

Ingredients:
- 6 fresh artichokes
- 6 anchovy fillets, chopped
- 4 garlic cloves, minced
- 2 tablespoons olive oil
- 1 cup breadcrumbs
- 1 tablespoon chopped parsley
- Salt and pepper to taste
- 1/4 cup white wine

Directions:
1. Cut the stem of each artichoke so that it sits flat on your chopping board then cut the top off and trim the outer leaves, cleaning the center as well.
2. In a bowl, mix the anchovy fillets, garlic, olive oil, breadcrumbs and parsley. Add salt and pepper to taste.
3. Top each artichoke with breadcrumb mixture and rub it well into the leaves.
4. Place the artichokes in your Crock Pot and pour in the white wine.
5. Cook on low settings for 6 hours.
6. Serve the artichokes warm or chilled.

Glazed Peanuts

Servings: 8
Cooking Time: 2 1/4 Hours

Ingredients:
- 2 pounds raw, whole peanuts
- 1/4 cup brown sugar
- 1/2 teaspoon garlic powder
- 2 tablespoons salt
- 1 tablespoon Cajun seasoning
- 1/2 teaspoon red pepper flakes
- 1/4 cup coconut oil

Directions:
1. Combine all the ingredients in your Crock Pot.
2. Cover and cook on high settings for 2 hours.
3. Serve chilled.

Parmesan Zucchini Frittata

Servings: 8
Cooking Time: 6 1/4 Hours

Ingredients:
- 2 zucchinis, finely sliced
- 2 garlic cloves, minced
- 1 teaspoon dried mint
- 1 teaspoon dried oregano
- 6 eggs
- 2 tablespoons plain yogurt
- 1 tablespoon chopped parsley
- 1/2 cup grated Parmesan
- Salt and pepper to taste

Directions:
1. Mix the zucchinis, garlic, dried mint and oregano in a Crock Pot.
2. Add salt and pepper to taste.
3. In a bowl, mix the eggs, yogurt, parsley and Parmesan.
4. Pour the egg mixture over the zucchinis and cover the pot with its lid.
5. Cook on low settings for 6 hours.
6. Serve the frittata sliced, warm or chilled.

Bacon Crab Dip

Servings: 20
Cooking Time: 2 1/4 Hours

Ingredients:
- 1 pound bacon, diced
- 1 cup cream cheese
- 1/2 cup grated Parmesan cheese
- 1 teaspoon Worcestershire sauce
- 1 teaspoon Dijon mustard
- 1 can crab meat, drained and shredded
- 1 teaspoon hot sauce

Directions:
1. Heat a skillet over medium flame and add the bacon. Sauté for 5 minutes until fat begins to drain out.
2. Transfer the bacon in a Crock Pot.
3. Stir in the remaining ingredients and cook on high settings for 2 hours.
4. Serve the dip warm or chilled.

Pizza Dip

Servings: 20
Cooking Time: 6 1/4 Hours

Ingredients:
- 1 pound spicy sausages, sliced
- 1/2 pound salami, diced
- 1 red bell pepper, cored and diced
- 1 yellow bell pepper, cored and sliced
- 1 onion, chopped
- 2 garlic cloves, minced
- 2 cups tomato sauce
- 1/2 cup grated Parmesan
- 1 cup shredded mozzarella
- 1/2 teaspoon dried basil
- 1/2 teaspoon dried oregano

Directions:
1. Layer all the ingredients in your Crock Pot.
2. Cook on low settings for 6 hours, mixing once during the cooking time to ensure an even distribution of ingredients.
3. Serve the dip warm.

Mixed Olive Dip

Servings: 10
Cooking Time: 1 3/4 Hours

Ingredients:
- 1 pound ground chicken
- 2 tablespoons olive oil
- 1 green bell pepper, cored and diced
- 1/2 cup Kalamata olives, pitted and chopped
- 1/2 cup green olives, chopped
- 1/2 cup black olives, pitted and chopped
- 1 cup green salsa
- 1/2 cup chicken stock
- 1 cup grated Cheddar cheese
- 1/2 cup shredded mozzarella

Directions:
1. Combine all the ingredients in your Crock Pot.
2. Cover with its lid and cook on high settings for 1 1/2 hours.
3. The dip is best served warm.

Cheesy Mushroom Dip

Servings: 16
Cooking Time: 4 1/4 Hours

Ingredients:
- 1 can condensed cream of mushroom soup
- 1 pound mushrooms, chopped
- 1 teaspoon Worcestershire sauce
- 1/4 cup evaporated milk
- 1/2 teaspoon chili powder
- 1 cup grated Cheddar cheese
- 1 cup grated Swiss cheese

Directions:
1. Mix the cream of mushroom soup, mushrooms, Worcestershire sauce, evaporated milk and chili powder in your Crock Pot.
2. Top with grated cheese and cook on low settings for 4 hours.
3. Serve the dip warm or re-heated.

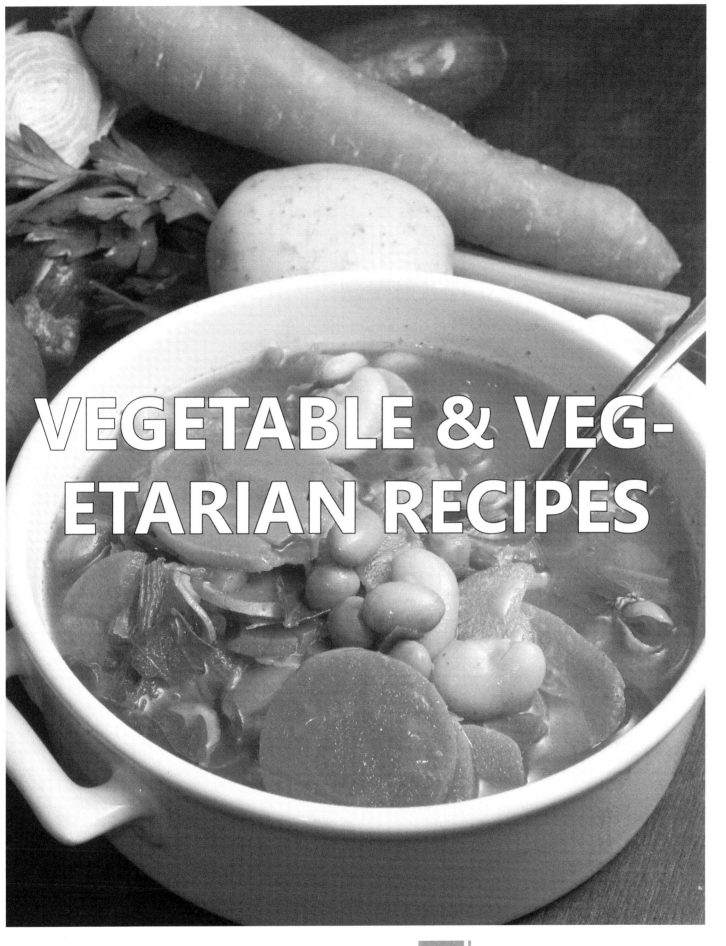

VEGETABLE & VEG-ETARIAN RECIPES

Zucchini Soup With Rosemary And Parmesan

Servings:6
Cooking Time: 3 Hours

Ingredients:
- 2 tablespoons olive oil
- 1 tablespoon butter
- 1 onion, chopped
- 1 teaspoon minced garlic
- 1 teaspoon Italian seasoning
- 4 teaspoons rosemary, chopped
- 2 pounds zucchini, chopped
- 8 cups vegetable stock
- Salt and pepper to taste
- 1 cup grated parmesan cheese

Directions:
1. Place all ingredients except for the parmesan cheese in the CrockPot.
2. Give a good stir.
3. Close the lid and cook on high for 3 hours or on low for 4 hours
4. Place inside a blender and pulse until smooth.
5. Serve with parmesan cheese on top.

Nutrition Info:
- Calories per serving: 172; Carbohydrates: 5.9g; Protein: 9.2g; Fat: 13.7g; Sugar: 0g; Sodium: 367mg; Fiber: 2.6g

Vegetable Bean Stew

Servings: 8
Cooking Time: 7 Hrs

Ingredients:
- ½ cup barley
- 1 cup black beans
- ¼ cup red beans
- 2 carrots, peeled and julienned
- 1 cup onion, chopped
- 1 cup tomato juice
- 2 potatoes, peeled and diced

- 1 tsp salt
- 1 tsp ground black pepper
- 4 cups of water
- 4 oz. tofu
- 1 tsp garlic powder
- 1 cup fresh cilantro

Directions:
1. Add black beans, red beans, and barley to the Crock Pot.
2. Stir in tomato juice, onion, garlic powder, black pepper, salt, and water.
3. Put the cooker's lid on and set the cooking time to 4 hours on High settings.
4. Add carrots, cilantro, and potatoes to the cooker.
5. Put the cooker's lid on and set the cooking time to 3 hours on Low settings.
6. Serve warm.

Nutrition Info:
- Per Serving: Calories 207, Total Fat 3.5g, Fiber 8g, Total Carbs 37.67g, Protein 8g

Green Peas Risotto

Servings: 6
Cooking Time: 3 Hrs 30 Minutes

Ingredients:
- 7 oz. Parmigiano-Reggiano
- 2 cup chicken broth
- 1 tsp olive oil
- 1 onion, chopped
- ½ cup green peas
- 1 garlic clove, peeled and sliced
- 2 cups long-grain rice
- ¼ cup dry wine
- 1 tsp salt
- 1 tsp ground black pepper
- 1 carrot, chopped
- 1 cup beef broth

Directions:
1. Layer a nonstick skillet with olive oil and place it over medium heat.
2. Stir in carrot and onion, then sauté for 3 minutes.

3. Transfer these veggies to the Crock Pot.

4. Add rice to the remaining oil to the skillet.

5. Stir cook for 1 minute then transfers the rice to the cooker.

6. Add garlic, dry wine, green peas, black pepper, beef broth, and chicken broth.

7. Put the cooker's lid on and set the cooking time to 3 hours on Low settings.

8. Add Parmigiano-Reggiano to the risotto.

9. Put the cooker's lid on and set the cooking time to 30 minutes on Low settings.

10. Serve warm.

Nutrition Info:
- Per Serving: Calories 268, Total Fat 3g, Fiber 4g, Total Carbs 53.34g, Protein 7g

Cauliflower Mac And Cheese

Servings:6
Cooking Time: 4 Hours

Ingredients:
- 1 large cauliflower, cut into small florets
- 2 tablespoons butter
- 1 cup heavy cream
- 2 ounces grass-fed cream cheese
- 1 ½ teaspoons Dijon mustard
- 1 ½ cup organic sharp cheddar cheese
- 1 tablespoon garlic powder
- ½ cup nutritional yeast
- Salt and pepper to taste

Directions:
1. Place all ingredients in the CrockPot.

2. Give a good stir.

3. Close the lid and cook on high for 3 hours or on low for 4 hours.

Nutrition Info:
- Calories per serving:329; Carbohydrates: 10.8g; Protein: 16.1g; Fat: 25.5g; Sugar: 0g; Sodium: 824mg; Fiber: 5.8g

Broccoli Egg Pie

Servings: 7
Cooking Time: 4 Hrs 25 Minutes

Ingredients:
- 7 oz. pie crust
- ¼ cup broccoli, chopped
- 1/3 cup sweet peas

- ¼ cup heavy cream
- 2 tbsp flour
- 3 eggs
- 4 oz. Romano cheese, shredded
- 1 tsp cilantro
- 1 tsp salt
- ¼ cup spinach, chopped
- 1 tomato, chopped

Directions:
1. Cover the base of your Crock Pot with a parchment sheet.

2. Spread the pie crust in the cooker and press it with your fingertips.

3. Mix chopped broccoli, sweet peas, flour, cream, salt, and cilantro in a bowl.

4. Beat eggs and add them to the cream mixture.

5. Stir in tomatoes and spinach to this mixture.

6. Spread this broccoli filling in the crust evenly

7. Put the cooker's lid on and set the cooking time to 4 hours on High settings.

8. Drizzle cheese over the quiche and cover it again.

9. Put the cooker's lid on and set the cooking time to 25 minutes on High settings.

10. Serve warm.

Nutrition Info:
- Per Serving: Calories 287, Total Fat 18.8g, Fiber 1g, Total Carbs 17.1g, Protein 11g

Shallot Saute

Servings:2
Cooking Time: 2.5 Hours

Ingredients:
- ½ cup carrot, grated
- 1 cup shallot, sliced
- 1 teaspoon ground turmeric
- ½ teaspoon salt
- 1 teaspoon garlic, diced
- ½ cup milk

Directions:
1. Put all ingredients in the Crock Pot.

2. Close the lid and cook the saute on High for 2 hours.

3. Then leave the cooked meal for 30 minutes to rest.

Nutrition Info:
- Per Serving: 105 calories, 4.4g protein, 20.3g carbohydrates, 1.5g fat, 0.9g fiber, 5mg cholesterol, 639mg sodium, 424mg potassium.

Creamy Keto Mash

Servings: 3
Cooking Time: 4 Hours

Ingredients:
- 1 cauliflower head, cut into florets
- 1 white onion, chopped
- 2 cloves of garlic, minced
- ¼ cup vegetable stock
- ¼ cup butter
- Salt and pepper to taste
- ½ cup cream cheese

Directions:
1. Place the all ingredients except for the cream cheese in the CrockPot.
2. Close the lid and cook on high for 3 hours or on low for 4 hours.
3. Place in the food processor and pour in the cream cheese. Pulse until slightly fine.
4. Garnish with chopped parsley if desired.

Nutrition Info:
- Calories per serving: 302; Carbohydrates: 7g; Protein: 3.7g; Fat: 28g; Sugar: 0g; Sodium: 771mg; Fiber: 3.8g

Quinoa Black Bean Chili

Servings: 4
Cooking Time: 3 Hrs

Ingredients:
- 15 oz. canned black beans, drained
- 2 and ¼ cups veggie stock
- ½ cup quinoa
- 14 oz. canned tomatoes, chopped
- ¼ cup red bell pepper, chopped
- 1 carrot, sliced
- ¼ cup green bell pepper, chopped
- 2 garlic cloves, minced
- ½ chili pepper, chopped
- ½ cup of corn
- 2 tsp chili powder
- 1 small yellow onion, chopped
- Salt and black pepper to the taste
- 1 tsp oregano, dried
- 1 tsp cumin, ground

Directions:
1. Add black beans and other ingredients to the Crock Pot.

2. Put the cooker's lid on and set the cooking time to 3 hours on High settings.
3. Serve warm.

Nutrition Info:
- Per Serving: Calories 291, Total Fat 7g, Fiber 4g, Total Carbs 28g, Protein 8g

Cream Of Mushroom Soup

Servings: 4
Cooking Time: 3 Hours

Ingredients:
- 1 tablespoons olive oil
- ½ cup onion, diced
- 20 ounces mushrooms, sliced
- 2 cups chicken broth
- 1 cup heavy cream

Directions:
1. In a skillet, heat the oil over medium flame and sauté the onions until translucent or slightly brown on the edges.
2. Transfer into the crockpot and add the mushrooms and chicken broth. Season with salt and pepper to taste.
3. Close the lid and cook on low for 6 hours or on high for 3 hours until the mushrooms are soft
4. Halfway before the cooking time ends, stir in the heavy cream.

Nutrition Info:
- Calories per serving: 229; Carbohydrates: 9g; Protein: 5g; Fat: 21g; Sugar:3 g; Sodium:214 mg; Fiber: 2g

Potato Balls

Servings: 6
Cooking Time: 1.5 Hours

Ingredients:
- 2 cups mashed potato
- 1 tablespoon coconut cream
- 3 tablespoons breadcrumbs
- 1 teaspoon dried dill
- 2 oz scallions, diced
- 1 egg, beaten
- 2 tablespoons flour
- ½ cup of coconut milk

Directions:
1. In the mixing bowl mix mashed potato with coco-

nut cream, breadcrumbs, dried dill, scallions, egg, and flour.

2. Make the potato balls and put them in the Crock Pot.

3. Add coconut milk and cook the meal on High for 1.5 hours.

Nutrition Info:
• Per Serving: 132 calories, 3.4g protein, 17.5g carbohydrates, 5.5g fat, 1.6g fiber, 28mg cholesterol, 273mg sodium, 287mg potassium.

Squash Noodles

Servings:4
Cooking Time: 4 Hours

Ingredients:
• 1-pound butternut squash, seeded, halved
• 1 tablespoon vegan butter
• 1 teaspoon salt
• ½ teaspoon garlic powder
• 3 cups of water

Directions:
1. Pour water in the Crock Pot.
2. Add butternut squash and close the lid.
3. Cook the vegetable on high for 4 hours.
4. Then drain water and shred the squash flesh with the help of the fork and transfer in the bowl.
5. Add garlic powder, salt, and butter. Mix the squash noodles.

Nutrition Info:
• Per Serving: 78 calories, 1.2g protein, 13.5g carbohydrates, 3g fat, 2.3g fiber, 8mg cholesterol, 612mg sodium, 406mg potassium

Mashed Turnips

Servings:6
Cooking Time: 7 Hours

Ingredients:
• 3-pounds turnip, chopped
• 3 cups of water
• 1 tablespoon vegan butter
• 1 tablespoon chives, chopped
• 2 oz Parmesan, grated

Directions:
1. Put turnips in the Crock Pot.
2. Add water and cook the vegetables on low for 7 hours.

3. Then drain water and mash the turnips.
4. Add chives, butter, and Parmesan.
5. Carefully stir the mixture until butter and Parmesan are melted.
6. Then add chives. Mix the mashed turnips again.

Nutrition Info:
• Per Serving: 162 calories, 8.6g protein, 15.1g carbohydrates, 8.1g fat, 4.1g fiber, 22mg cholesterol, 475mg sodium, 490mg potassium.

Sauteed Garlic

Servings:4
Cooking Time: 6 Hours

Ingredients:
• 10 oz garlic cloves, peeled
• 2 tablespoons lemon juice
• 1 teaspoon ground black pepper
• 1 cup of water
• 1 tablespoon vegan butter
• 1 bay leaf

Directions:
1. Put all ingredients in the Crock Pot.
2. Close the lid and cook the garlic on Low for 6 hours.

Nutrition Info:
• Per Serving: 135 calories, 4.7g protein, 24.1g carbohydrates, 3.3g fat, 1.7g fiber, 8mg cholesterol, 36mg sodium, 303mg potassium

Cauliflower Rice

Servings:6
Cooking Time: 2 Hours

Ingredients:
• 4 cups cauliflower, shredded
• 1 cup vegetable stock
• 1 cup of water
• 1 tablespoon cream cheese
• 1 teaspoon dried oregano

Directions:
1. Put all ingredients in the Crock Pot.
2. Close the lid and cook the cauliflower rice on High for 2 hours.

Nutrition Info:
• Per Serving: 25 calories, 0.8g protein, 3.9g carbohydrates, 0.8g fat, 1.8g fiber, 2mg cholesterol, 153mg sodium, 211mg potassium

Teriyaki Kale

Servings:6
Cooking Time: 30 Minutes

Ingredients:
- 5 cups kale, roughly chopped
- 1/2 cup teriyaki sauce
- 1 teaspoon sesame seeds
- 1 cup of water
- 1 teaspoon garlic powder
- 2 tablespoons coconut oil

Directions:
1. Melt the coconut oil and mix it with garlic powder, water, sesame seeds, and teriyaki sauce.
2. Pour the liquid in the Crock Pot.
3. Add kale and close the lid.
4. Cook the kale on High for 30 minutes.
5. Serve the kale with a small amount of teriyaki liquid.

Nutrition Info:
- Per Serving: 92 calories, 3.3g protein, 10g carbohydrates, 4.8g fat, 1g fiber, 0mg cholesterol, 945mg sodium, 336mg potassium.

Zucchini Basil Soup

Servings:8
Cooking Time: 3 Hours

Ingredients:
- 9 cups zucchini, diced
- 2 cups white onions, chopped
- 4 cups vegetable broth
- 8 cloves of garlic, minced
- 1 cup basil leaves
- 4 tablespoons olive oil
- Salt and pepper to taste

Directions:
1. Place the ingredients in the CrockPot.
2. Give a good stir.
3. Close the lid and cook on high for 2 hours or on low for 3 hours.
4. Once cooked, transfer into a blender and pulse until smooth.

Nutrition Info:
- Calories per serving: 93; Carbohydrates: 5.4g; Protein: 1.3g; Fat: 11.6g; Sugar: 0g; Sodium: 322mg; Fiber: 4.2g

Miso Asparagus

Servings:2
Cooking Time: 2.5 Hours

Ingredients:
- 1 teaspoon miso paste
- 1 cup of water
- 1 tablespoon fish sauce
- 10 oz asparagus, chopped
- 1 teaspoon avocado oil

Directions:
1. Mix miso paste with water and pour in the Crock Pot.
2. Add fish sauce, asparagus, and avocado oil.
3. Close the lid and cook the meal on High for 2.5 hours.

Nutrition Info:
- Per Serving: 40 calories, 3.9g protein, 6.7g carbohydrates, 0.6g fat, 3.2g fiber, 0mg cholesterol, 808mg sodium, 327mg potassium.

Vegan Pepper Bowl

Servings:4
Cooking Time: 3.5 Hours

Ingredients:
- 2 cups bell pepper, sliced
- 1 tablespoon olive oil
- 1 tablespoon apple cider vinegar
- 4 tablespoons water
- 5 oz tofu, chopped
- ½ cup of coconut milk
- 1 teaspoon curry powder

Directions:
1. Put the sliced bell peppers in the Crock Pot.
2. Sprinkle them with olive oil, apple cider vinegar, and water.
3. Close the lid and cook the vegetables on low for 3 hours.
4. Meanwhile, mix curry powder with coconut milk. Put the tofu in the curry mixture and leave for 15 minutes.
5. Add the tofu and all remaining curry mixture in the Crock Pot. Gently mix it and cook for 30 minutes on low.

Nutrition Info:
- Per Serving: 145 calories, 4.3g protein, 7.1g carbohydrates, 12.4g fat, 2g fiber, 0mg cholesterol, 11mg

sodium, 254mg potassium.

Cinnamon Banana Sandwiches

Servings: 4
Cooking Time: 2 Hrs

Ingredients:
- 2 bananas, peeled and sliced
- 8 oz. French toast slices, frozen
- 1 tbsp peanut butter
- ¼ tsp ground cinnamon
- 5 oz. Cheddar cheese, sliced
- ¼ tsp turmeric

Directions:
1. Layer half of the French toast slices with peanut butter.
2. Whisk cinnamon with turmeric and drizzle over the peanut butter layer.
3. Place the banana slice and cheese slices over the toasts.
4. Now place the remaining French toast slices on top.
5. Place these banana sandwiches in the Crock Pot.
6. Put the cooker's lid on and set the cooking time to 2 hours on High settings.
7. Serve.

Nutrition Info:
- Per Serving: Calories 248, Total Fat 7.5g, Fiber 2g, Total Carbs 36.74g, Protein 10g

Sweet Pineapple Tofu

Servings:2
Cooking Time: 15 Minutes

Ingredients:
- 1/3 cup pineapple juice
- 1 teaspoon brown sugar
- 1 teaspoon ground cinnamon
- ¼ teaspoon ground cardamom
- 7 oz firm tofu, chopped
- 1 teaspoon olive oil

Directions:
1. Put tofu in the mixing bowl.
2. Then sprinkle it with pineapple juice, brown sugar, ground cinnamon, cardamom, and olive oil. Carefully mix the tofu and leave it for 10-15 minutes.
3. Then transfer the tofu mixture in the Crock Pot and close the lid.
4. Cook it on High for 15 minutes.

Nutrition Info:
- Per Serving: 121 calories, 8.4g protein, 9.6g carbohydrates, 6.6g fat, 1.7g fiber, 0mg cholesterol, 13mg sodium, 211mg potassium.

Vegan Kofte

Servings:4
Cooking Time: 4 Hours

Ingredients:
- 2 eggplants, peeled, boiled
- 1 teaspoon minced garlic
- 1 teaspoon ground cumin
- ¼ teaspoon minced ginger
- ½ cup chickpeas, canned
- 3 tablespoons breadcrumbs
- 1/3 cup water
- 1 tablespoon coconut oil

Directions:
1. Blend the eggplants until smooth.
2. Add minced garlic, ground cumin, minced ginger, chickpeas, and blend the mixture until smooth.
3. Transfer it in the mixing bowl. Add breadcrumbs.
4. Make the small koftes and put them in the Crock Pot.
5. Add coconut oil and close the lid.
6. Cook the meal on Low for 4 hours.

Nutrition Info:
- Per Serving: 212 calories, 8.3g protein, 35.5g carbohydrates, 5.8g fat, 14.3g fiber, 0mg cholesterol, 50mg sodium, 870mg potassium.

Beet And Capers Salad

Servings:4
Cooking Time: 4 Hours

Ingredients:
- 2 teaspoons capers
- 1 cup lettuce, chopped
- 2 oz walnuts, chopped
- 1 tablespoon lemon juice
- 1 tablespoon sunflower oil
- 1 teaspoon flax seeds
- 3 cups of water
- 2 cups beets, peeled

Directions:
1. Pour water in the Crock Pot and add beets. Cook them on High for 4 hours.

2. Then drain water, cool the beets and chop.
3. Put the chopped beets in the salad bowl.
4. Add capers, lettuce, walnuts, lemon juice, sunflower oil, and flax seeds.
5. Carefully mix the salad.

Nutrition Info:
• Per Serving: 162 calories, 5.1g protein, 10.6g carbohydrates, 12.3g fat, 3g fiber, 0mg cholesterol, 115mg sodium, 365mg potassium.

Paprika Baby Carrot

Servings:2
Cooking Time: 2.5 Hours

Ingredients:
• 1 tablespoon ground paprika
• 2 cups baby carrot
• 1 teaspoon cumin seeds
• 1 cup of water
• 1 teaspoon vegan butter

Directions:
1. Pour water in the Crock Pot.
2. Add baby carrot, cumin seeds, and ground paprika.
3. Close the lid and cook the carrot on High for 2.5 hours.
4. Then drain water, add butter, and shake the vegetables.

Nutrition Info:
• Per Serving: 60 calories, 1.6g protein, 8.6g carbohydrates, 2.7g fat, 4.2g fiber, 5mg cholesterol, 64mg sodium, 220mg potassium.

Sautéed Endives

Servings:4
Cooking Time: 40 Minutes

Ingredients:
• 1-pound endives, roughly chopped
• ½ cup of water
• 1 tablespoon avocado oil
• 1 teaspoon garlic, diced
• 2 tablespoons coconut cream

Directions:
1. Pour water in the Crock Pot.
2. Add endives and garlic.
3. Close the lid and cook them on High for 30 minutes.
4. Then add coconut cream and avocado oil.

5. Cook the endives for 10 minutes more.

Nutrition Info:
• Per Serving: 42 calories, 1.9g protein, 4.4g carbohydrates, 2.4g fat, 3.7g fiber, 6mg cholesterol, 41mg sodium, 376mg potassium.

Oregano Cheese Pie

Servings: 6
Cooking Time: 3.5 Hrs

Ingredients:
• 1 tsp baking soda
• 1 tbsp lemon juice
• 1 cup flour
• 1 cup milk
• 1 tsp salt
• 5 oz. Cheddar cheese, shredded
• 5 oz. Parmesan cheese, shredded
• 2 eggs
• ½ tsp oregano
• 1/3 tsp olive oil

Directions:
1. Sift flour with salt, oregano, baking soda and shredded cheese in a bowl.
2. Beat eggs with lemon juice and milk in a separate bowl.
3. Gradually stir in flour mixture and mix using a hand mixer until it forms a smooth dough.
4. Layer the base of Crock Pot with olive oil and spread the dough in the cooker.
5. Put the cooker's lid on and set the cooking time to 3 hours 30 minutes on High settings.
6. Serve.

Nutrition Info:
• Per Serving: Calories 288, Total Fat 13.7g, Fiber 1g, Total Carbs 24.23g, Protein 16g

Sweet And Tender Squash

Servings:4
Cooking Time: 8 Hours

Ingredients:
• 2-pound butternut squash, chopped
• 1 tablespoon ground cinnamon
• ½ teaspoon ground ginger
• 1 tablespoon sugar
• ½ cup of water

Directions:

1. Mix butternut squash with ground cinnamon, ground ginger, and sugar. Leave the vegetables for 10-15 minutes.
2. Then transfer them in the Crock Pot. Add remaining butternut squash juice and water.
3. Close the lid and cook the squash on Low for 8 hours.

Nutrition Info:
• Per Serving: 118 calories, 2.4g protein, 31g carbohydrates, 0.3g fat, 5.5g fiber, 0mg cholesterol, 10mg sodium, 809mg potassium.

Cashew And Tofu Casserole

Servings:4
Cooking Time: 3.5 Hours

Ingredients:
• 1 oz cashews, crushed
• 6 oz firm tofu, chopped
• 1 cup broccoli, chopped
• 1 red onion, sliced
• 1 tablespoon avocado oil
• ¼ cup of soy sauce
• ¼ cup maple syrup
• 1 tablespoon cornstarch
• ½ cup of water
• 1 teaspoon garlic powder

Directions:
1. Pour the avocado oil in the Crock Pot.
2. Then sprinkle the broccoli with garlic powder and put it in the Crock Pot.
3. Add cornstarch.
4. After this, add maple syrup, soy sauce, onion, and tofu.
5. Add cashews and water.
6. Close the lid and cook the casserole on Low for 3.5 hours.

Nutrition Info:
• Per Serving: 164 calories, 6.7g protein, 24g carbohydrates, 5.7g fat, 2.1g fiber, 0mg cholesterol, 917mg sodium, 309mg potassium.

Rice Stuffed Apple Cups

Servings: 4
Cooking Time: 6 Hrs

Ingredients:
• 4 red apples
• 1 cup white rice
• 3 tbsp raisins
• 1 onion, diced
• 7 tbsp water
• 1 tsp salt
• 1 tsp curry powder
• 4 tsp sour cream

Directions:
1. Remove the seeds and half of the flesh from the center of the apples to make apple cups.
2. Toss onion with white rice, curry powder, salt, and raisin in a separate bowl.
3. Divide this rice-raisins mixture into the apple cups.
4. Pour water into the Crock Pot and place the stuffed cups in it.
5. Top the apples with sour cream.
6. Put the cooker's lid on and set the cooking time to 6 hours on Low settings.
7. Serve.

Nutrition Info:
• Per Serving: Calories 317, Total Fat 1.3g, Fiber 7g, Total Carbs 71.09g, Protein 4g

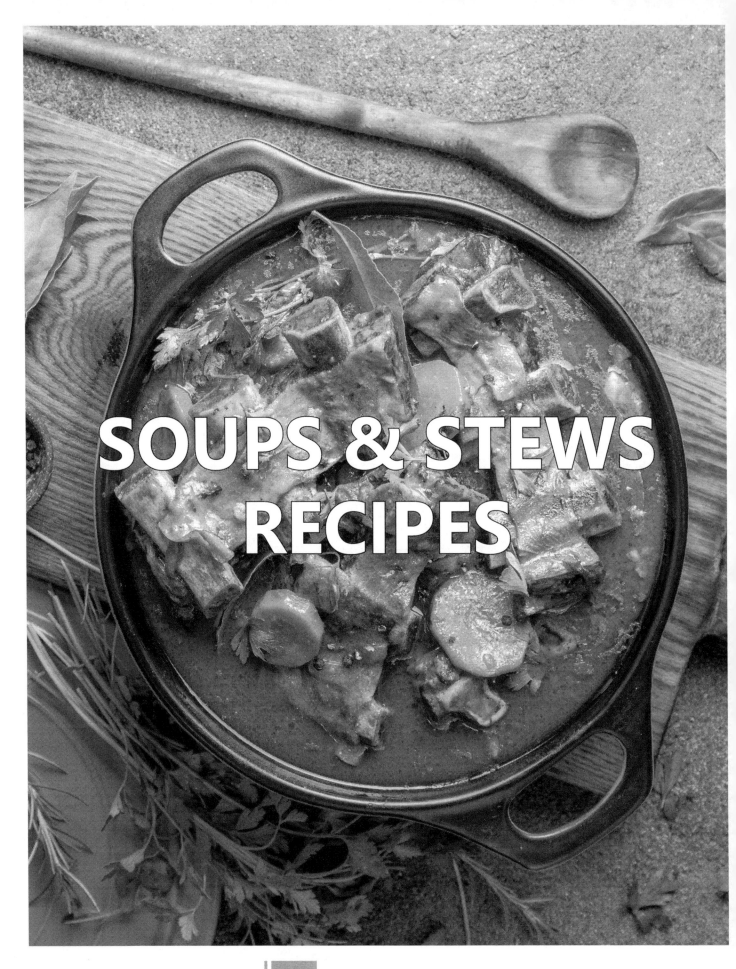

SOUPS & STEWS RECIPES

Barley Soup

Servings:5
Cooking Time: 8 Hours

Ingredients:
- ¼ cup barley
- 5 cups chicken stock
- 4 oz pork tenderloin, chopped
- 1 tablespoon dried cilantro
- 1 tablespoon tomato paste
- 3 oz carrot, grated
- ½ cup heavy cream

Directions:
1. Put pork tenderloin in the Crock Pot.
2. Add barley, chicken stock, tomato paste, carrot, and heavy cream.
3. Carefully stir the soup mixture and close the lid.
4. Cook it on Low for 8 hours.

Nutrition Info:
- Per Serving: 126 calories, 8.3g protein, 10.1g carbohydrates, 6g fat, 2.2g fiber, 33mg cholesterol, 797mg sodium, 249mg potassium.

Snow Peas Soup

Servings:4
Cooking Time: 3.5 Hours

Ingredients:
- 1 tablespoon chives, chopped
- 1 teaspoon ground ginger
- 8 oz salmon fillet, chopped
- 5 oz bamboo shoots, canned, chopped
- 2 cups snow peas
- 1 teaspoon hot sauce
- 5 cups of water

Directions:
1. Put bamboo shoots in the Crock Pot.
2. Add ground ginger, salmon, snow peas, and water.
3. Close the lid and cook the soup for 3 hours on high.
4. Then add hot sauce and chives. Stir the soup carefully and cook for 30 minutes on high.

Nutrition Info:
- Per Serving: 120 calories, 14.6g protein, 7.9g carbohydrates, 3.8g fat, 3.1g fiber, 25mg cholesterol, 70mg sodium, 612mg potassium

Provencal Beef Soup

Servings: 8
Cooking Time: 7 1/4 Hours

Ingredients:
- 2 tablespoons olive oil
- 1 pound beef roast, cubed
- 1 sweet onion, chopped
- 1 garlic clove, chopped
- 2 carrots, sliced
- 1 celery stalk, sliced
- 1 can diced tomatoes
- 1 cup beef stock
- 1 cup red wine
- 4 cups water
- 1/2 teaspoon dried thyme
- 1 bay leaf
- Salt and pepper to taste

Directions:
1. Heat the oil in a skillet and stir in the beef roast. Cook on all sides for a few minutes then transfer the beef in a Crock Pot.
2. Add the remaining ingredients and adjust the taste with salt and pepper.
3. Cook on low settings for 7 hours.
4. Serve the soup warm or chilled.

Beef Bacon Barley Soup

Servings: 8
Cooking Time: 8 1/2 Hours

Ingredients:
- 4 bacon slices, chopped
- 1 pound beef steak, cubed
- 1/2 teaspoon smoked paprika
- 1 medium onion, chopped
- 4 small potatoes, peeled and cubed

- 1 cup baby carrots, halved
- 1 cup frozen sweet corn
- 1 cup fire roasted tomatoes
- 1/2 cup pearl barley, rinsed
- 2 cups beef stock
- 4 cups water
- 1/2 teaspoon dried basil
- 1/2 teaspoon dried oregano
- Salt and pepper to taste

Directions:
1. Heat a skillet over medium flame and add the bacon. Cook until crisp then stir in the beef. Cook on all sides until golden for about 5 minutes. Transfer in your Crock Pot.
2. Add the remaining ingredients and season with salt and pepper.
3. Cook the soup on low settings for 8 hours.
4. Serve the soup warm.

Creamy Spinach Tortellini Soup

Servings: 8
Cooking Time: 6 1/4 Hours

Ingredients:
- 1 chicken breast, diced
- 1 tablespoon olive oil
- 2 shallots, chopped
- 2 garlic cloves, chopped
- 2 cups tomato sauce
- 4 cups chicken stock
- 1 can condensed mushroom soup
- 2 cups sliced mushrooms
- 1 cup water
- 8 oz. spinach tortellini
- Salt and pepper to taste

Directions:
1. Heat the oil in a skillet and add the chicken. Cook on all sides for 5 minutes then transfer in your Crock Pot.
2. Add the remaining ingredients and continue cooking on low settings for 6 hours.
3. The soup is best served warm, either fresh or re-heated.

French Soup

Servings:5
Cooking Time: 7 Hours

Ingredients:
- 5 oz Gruyere cheese, shredded
- 2 cups of water
- 2 cups chicken stock
- 2 cups white onion, diced
- ½ teaspoon cayenne pepper
- ½ cup heavy cream

Directions:
1. Pour chicken stock, water, and heavy cream in the Crock Pot.
2. Add onion, cayenne pepper, and close the lid.
3. Cook the ingredients on high for 4 hours.
4. When the time is finished, open the lid, stir the mixture, and add cheese.
5. Carefully mix the soup and cook it on Low for 3 hours.

Nutrition Info:
- Per Serving: 181 calories, 9.5g protein, 5.1g carbohydrates, 13.9g fat, 1g fiber, 48mg cholesterol, 410mg sodium, 110mg potassium.

Zucchini Soup

Servings: 6
Cooking Time: 2 1/4 Hours

Ingredients:
- 1 pound Italian sausages, sliced
- 2 celery stalks, sliced
- 2 zucchinis, cubed
- 2 large potatoes, peeled and cubed
- 2 yellow bell peppers, cored and diced
- 2 carrots, sliced
- 1 shallot, chopped
- 3 cups water
- 2 cups vegetable stock
- 1/2 teaspoon dried oregano
- 1/2 teaspoon dried basil
- 1/4 teaspoon garlic powder
- Salt and pepper to taste
- 2 tablespoons chopped parsley

Directions:
1. Combine the sausages, celery stalks, zucchinis, potatoes, bell peppers, carrots, shallot, water, stock and seasoning in your Crock Pot.

2. Add salt and pepper to taste and cook on high settings for 2 hours.
3. When done, stir in the parsley and serve the soup warm.

Spiced Creamy Pumpkin Soup

Servings: 6
Cooking Time: 5 1/4 Hours

Ingredients:
- 1 shallot, chopped
- 2 carrots, sliced
- 2 garlic cloves, chopped
- 2 tablespoons olive oil
- 1 medium sugar pumpkin, peeled and cubed
- 2 cups chicken stock
- 2 cups water
- 1 thyme sprig
- Salt and pepper to taste
- 1/2 cinnamon stick
- 1 star anise
- 1/2 teaspoon cumin powder
- 1/4 teaspoon chili powder

Directions:
1. Combine the shallot, carrots, garlic and olive oil in a skillet. Cook for 5 minutes until softened.
2. Transfer in your Crock Pot and add the remaining ingredients, including the spices.
3. Cook on low settings for 5 hours then remove the cinnamon, thyme sprig and star anise and puree the soup with an immersion blender.
4. The soup can be served either warm or chilled.

Mexican Style Stew

Servings:6
Cooking Time: 6 Hours

Ingredients:
- 1 cup corn kernels
- 1 cup green peas
- ¼ cup white rice
- 4 cups chicken stock
- 1 teaspoon taco seasoning
- 1 teaspoon dried cilantro
- 1 tablespoon butter

Directions:
1. Put butter and wild rice in the Crock Pot.
2. Then add corn kernels, green peas, chicken stock, taco seasoning, and dried cilantro.

3. Close the lid and cook the stew on Low for 6 hours.

Nutrition Info:
- Per Serving: 97 calories, 3.2g protein, 15.6g carbohydrates, 2.7g fat, 2g fiber, 5mg cholesterol, 599mg sodium, 148mg potassium.

Asparagus Crab Soup

Servings: 6
Cooking Time: 2 1/4 Hours

Ingredients:
- 1 tablespoon olive oil
- 1 shallot, chopped
- 1 celery stalk, sliced
- 1 bunch asparagus, trimmed and chopped
- 1 cup green peas
- 1 cup chicken stock
- 2 cups water
- Salt and pepper to taste
- 1 can crab meat, drained

Directions:
1. Heat the oil in a skillet and add the shallot and celery. Sauté for 2 minutes until softened then transfer in your Crock Pot.
2. Add the asparagus, green peas, stock and water and season with salt and pepper.
3. Cook on high settings for 2 hours.
4. When done, puree the soup with an immersion blender until creamy.
5. Pour the soup into serving bowls and top with crab meat.
6. Serve the soup right away.

Beef Mushroom Soup

Servings: 8
Cooking Time: 8 1/2 Hours

Ingredients:
- 1 pound beef roast, cubed
- 2 tablespoons canola oil
- 1 sweet onion, chopped
- 2 garlic cloves, chopped
- 1 pound mushrooms, sliced
- 1 can fire roasted tomatoes
- 2 cups beef stock
- 5 cups water
- 1 bay leaf
- 1 thyme sprig
- 1/2 teaspoon caraway seeds

- Salt and pepper to taste

Directions:
1. Heat the oil in a skillet and stir in the beef roast. Cook on all sides for a few minutes then transfer in your Crock Pot.
2. Add the onion, garlic, mushrooms, tomatoes, stock and water, as well as bay leaf and thyme sprig, plus the caraway seeds.
3. Season with salt and pepper and cook on low settings for 8 hours.
4. The soup is best served warm.

Chicken Pearl Barley Soup

Servings: 8
Cooking Time: 6 1/2 Hours

Ingredients:
- 3 chicken breasts, cubed
- 2 tablespoons olive oil
- 1 teaspoon dried oregano
- 1/2 teaspoon paprika
- 1 large sweet onion, chopped
- 2 carrots, sliced
- 2 celery stalks, sliced
- 2 tomatoes, peeled and diced
- 2 potatoes, peeled and cubed
- 1/2 cup pearl barley
- 2 cups chicken stock
- 4 cups water
- Salt and pepper to taste
- 2 tablespoons chopped parsley

Directions:
1. Heat the oil in a skillet and add the chicken. Cook on all sides for a few minutes until golden then transfer in your Crock Pot.
2. Add the oregano, paprika, onion, carrots, celery, tomatoes, potatoes, pearl barley, water, chicken stock, salt and pepper.
3. Cook on low settings for 6 hours.
4. When done, stir in the parsley and serve the soup warm.

Ham White Bean Soup

Servings: 6
Cooking Time: 2 1/4 Hours

Ingredients:
- 1 tablespoon olive oil
- 4 oz. ham, diced

- 1 sweet onion, chopped
- 2 garlic cloves, chopped
- 1 yellow bell pepper, cored and diced
- 1 red bell pepper, cored and diced
- 1 carrot, diced
- 1 cup diced tomatoes
- 1 can (15 oz.) white beans, drained
- 2 cups chicken stock
- 3 cups water
- Salt and pepper to taste

Directions:
1. Heat the oil in a skillet and add the ham. Cook for 2 minutes then stir in the onion and garlic. Sauté for 2 additional minutes.
2. Transfer the mixture in your Crock Pot and stir in the remaining ingredients.
3. Adjust the taste with salt and pepper and cook on high settings for 2 hours.
4. Serve the soup warm or chilled.

Crock-pot Clam Chowder

Servings: 8
Cooking Time: 6 Hours

Ingredients:
- 1 cup chopped onion
- 13 slices thick cut bacon
- 1 cup celery, chopped
- 2 cups chicken broth
- 2 cups heavy whipping cream
- 1 teaspoon thyme, ground
- 1 teaspoon sea salt
- 1 teaspoon pepper

Directions:
1. Cook the bacon until crispy and reserve the bacon grease in pan. Chop celery and onion. Place celery and onion in bacon grease and cook until soft; add grease to Crock-Pot along with veggies. Once veggies are soft, add them to the Crock-Pot and all other ingredients. Cover and cook on LOW for 6 hours.

Nutrition Info:
- Calories: 427, Total Fat: 33 g, Cholesterol: 252 mg, Sodium: 1636 mg, Potassium: 107 mg, Carbohydrates: 5 g, Dietary Fiber: 0 g, Sugars: 0 g, Protein: 27 g

Summer Squash Chickpea Soup

Servings: 6
Cooking Time: 2 1/2 Hours

Ingredients:

- 1 sweet onion, chopped
- 1 garlic clove, chopped
- 1 carrot, diced
- 1 celery stalk, sliced
- 2 summer squashes, cubed
- 1 can (15 oz.) chickpeas, drained
- 2 cups chicken stock
- 3 cups water
- 1 cup diced tomatoes
- 1 bay leaf
- 1 thyme sprig
- Salt and pepper to taste
- 1 lemon, juiced
- 1 tablespoon chopped cilantro
- 1 tablespoon chopped parsley

Directions:

1. Combine the onion, garlic, celery, carrot, summer squash, chickpeas, stock and water in your Crock Pot.
2. Add the tomatoes, bay leaf, thyme, salt and pepper and cook on high settings for 2 hours.
3. When done, stir in the lemon juice, parsley and cilantro and serve the soup warm.

Garlicky Chicken Soup

Servings: 6
Cooking Time: 6 1/4 Hours

Ingredients:

- 1 large chicken breast (bone in)
- 1 cup chicken stock
- 6 cups water
- 2 carrots, diced
- 1 sweet onion, chopped
- 1 parsnip, diced
- 1/2 celery root, peeled and diced
- Salt and pepper to taste
- 1 cup sour cream
- 2 egg yolks
- 4 garlic cloves, minced
- 2 tablespoons chopped parsley

Directions:

1. Combine the chicken breast, stock, water, carrots, onion, parsnip and celery in your Crock Pot.
2. Add salt and pepper to taste and cook on low settings for 6 hours.
3. When done, remove the chicken breast and place aside.
4. In a small bowl, mix the sour cream, egg yolks and garlic then pour this mixture over the hot soup. Mix well and stir in the parsley.
5. Remove the meat off the bone and shred it finely. Add it into the soup.
6. Serve the soup right away.

Orange Salmon Soup

Servings: 8
Cooking Time: 2 1/4 Hours

Ingredients:

- 1 sweet onion, chopped
- 1 garlic clove, chopped
- 1 celery stalk, sliced
- 1 small fennel bulb, sliced
- 1 cup diced tomatoes
- 3 salmon fillets, cubed
- 2 cups vegetable stock
- 3 cups water
- 1 lemon, juiced
- 1 orange, juiced
- 1/2 teaspoon grated orange zest
- Salt and pepper to taste

Directions:

1. Combine the onion, garlic, celery, fennel bulb, tomatoes, salmon, stock and water in your Crock Pot.
2. Add the remaining ingredients and season with salt and pepper.
3. Cook on high settings for 2 hours.
4. Serve the soup warm or chilled.

Creamy Edamame Soup

Servings: 6
Cooking Time: 2 1/4 Hours

Ingredients:

- 1 tablespoon olive oil
- 2 shallots, chopped
- 2 garlic cloves, chopped
- 1 large potato, peeled and cubed
- 1 celery root, peeled and cubed
- 1 pound frozen edamame
- Salt and pepper to taste
- 2 cups chicken stock
- 1 cup water

- 1/4 teaspoon dried oregano
- 1/4 teaspoon dried marjoram

Directions:

1. Heat the oil in a skillet and stir in the shallots and garlic. Sauté for 2 minutes until softened then transfer in your Crock Pot.
2. Add the remaining ingredients and season with salt and pepper.
3. Cook on high settings for 2 hours.
4. When done, puree the soup with an immersion blender until creamy.
5. Serve the soup right away.

Pumpkin Hearty Soup

Servings: 10
Cooking Time: 6 1/4 Hours

Ingredients:

- 2 tablespoons olive oil
- 2 shallots, chopped
- 2 garlic cloves, chopped
- 1 red chili, seeded and chopped
- 1/4 teaspoon grated ginger
- 2 tablespoons tomato paste
- 1 can diced tomatoes
- 1 can (15 oz.) black beans, drained
- 2 cups pumpkin cubes
- 2 cups water
- 3 cups vegetable stock
- 1 bay leaf
- Salt and pepper to taste
- 1/2 cinnamon stick
- 1/4 teaspoon cumin powder

Directions:

1. Heat the oil in a skillet or saucepan and add the shallots, garlic, red chili and ginger. Cook for 3-4 minutes then transfer in your Crock Pot.
2. Add the tomato paste, tomatoes, black beans and pumpkin, as well as the water, stock, bay leaf, cinnamon and cumin.
3. Adjust the taste with salt and cook on low settings for 6 hours.
4. Serve the soup warm and fresh.

Beef Cabbage Soup

Servings: 8
Cooking Time: 7 1/2 Hours

Ingredients:

- 1 pound beef roast, cubed
- 2 tablespoons olive oil
- 1 sweet onion, chopped
- 1 carrot, grated
- 1 small cabbage head, shredded
- 1 can (15 oz.) diced tomatoes
- 2 cups beef stock
- 2 cups water
- 1/2 teaspoon cumin seeds
- Salt and pepper to taste

Directions:

1. Heat the oil in a skillet and add the beef roast. Cook for 5-6 minutes on all sides then transfer the meat in your Crock Pot.
2. Add the remaining ingredients and season with salt and pepper.
3. Cook on low settings for 7 hours.
4. Serve the cabbage soup warm.

Spicy Black Bean Soup

Servings: 6
Cooking Time: 6 1/4 Hours

Ingredients:

- 1 tablespoon olive oil
- 1 shallot, chopped
- 1 carrot, diced
- 2 jalapeno peppers, chopped
- 2 cups chicken stock
- 1 can (15 oz.) black beans, drained
- 4 cups water
- 1/2 teaspoon chili powder
- 1/2 teaspoon cumin powder
- 1/2 cup diced tomatoes
- Salt and pepper to taste
- 1/2 cup sour cream

Directions:

1. Combine the olive oil, shallot, carrot, jalapeno peppers, stock, beans, water and spices in your Crock Pot.
2. Add salt and pepper to taste and cook on low settings for 6 hours.
3. Cook on low settings for6 hours.
4. Serve the soup warm, topped with sour cream.

Leek Potato Soup

Servings: 8
Cooking Time: 6 1/2 Hours

Ingredients:
- 4 leeks, sliced
- 1 tablespoon olive oil
- 4 bacon slices, chopped
- 1 celery stalk, sliced
- 4 large potatoes, peeled and cubed
- 2 cups chicken stock
- 3 cups water
- 1 bay leaf
- Salt and pepper to taste
- 1/4 teaspoon cayenne pepper
- 1/4 teaspoon smoked paprika
- 1 thyme sprig
- 1 rosemary sprig

Directions:
1. Heat the oil in a skillet and add the bacon. Cook until crisp then stir in the leeks.
2. Sauté for 5 minutes until softened then transfer in your Crock Pot.
3. Add the remaining ingredients and cook on low settings for about 6 hours.
4. Serve the soup warm.

Celery Soup With Ham

Servings:8
Cooking Time: 5 Hours

Ingredients:
- 8 oz ham, chopped
- 8 cups chicken stock
- 1 teaspoon white pepper
- ½ teaspoon cayenne pepper
- 2 cups celery stalk, chopped
- ½ cup corn kernels

Directions:
1. Put all ingredients in the Crock Pot and gently stir.
2. Close the lid and cook the soup on High for 5 hours.
3. When the soup is cooked, cool it to the room temperature and ladle into the bowls.

Nutrition Info:
- Per Serving: 69 calories, 5.9g protein, 4.6g carbohydrates, 3.2g fat, 1.1g fiber, 16mg cholesterol, 1155mg sodium, 193mg potassium.

Minced Beef & Vegetable Soup

Servings: 6 (8.2 Ounces Per Serving)
Cooking Time: 8 Hours And 15 Minutes

Ingredients:
- 1 ½ lbs. lean minced meat (beef)
- 1 sweet potato, cubed
- 2 sticks of celery, sliced
- 3 carrots, sliced
- 2 green onions, finely sliced
- 4 tablespoons tomato paste, sugar-free and low sodium
- 1 ½ cups water
- Salt and black pepper to taste
- ½ cup green beans, chopped

Directions:
1. In a large skillet, sauté the minced meat over medium-high heat. Drain the fat and set aside. Layer the bottom of Crock-Pot with potatoes. Spread the celery and green beans on top of potatoes, then spread a layer of meat on top of celery. Season with salt and pepper. Add chopped carrots and onions. In a bowl, mix tomato paste and water and pour into Crock Pot over remaining ingredients. Cover and cook for 6-8 hours. Serve hot.

Nutrition Info:
- Calories: 323.8, Total Fat: 25.12 g, Saturated Fat: 9.42 g, Cholesterol: 64.86 mg, Sodium: 107.4 mg, Potassium: 586.28 mg, Total Carbohydrates: 8.05 g, Fiber: 2.17 g, Sugar: 3.29 g, Protein: 13.35 g

Vegetable Chickpea Soup

Servings: 6
Cooking Time: 6 1/2 Hours

Ingredients:
- 2/3 cup dried chickpeas, rinsed
- 2 cups chicken stock
- 4 cups water
- 1 celery stalk, sliced
- 1 carrot, diced
- 1 shallot, chopped
- 2 ripe tomatoes, peeled and diced
- 1 red bell pepper, cored and diced
- 1 potato, peeled and diced
- 1 tablespoon lemon juice
- Salt and pepper to taste

Directions:

1. Combine all the ingredients in your Crock Pot.
2. Add salt and pepper to taste and cook on low settings for 6 hours.
3. Serve the soup warm and fresh.

Pesto Chicken Soup

Servings: 6
Cooking Time: 6 1/4 Hours

Ingredients:
- 1 chicken breast, cubed
- 1 shallot, chopped
- 1 garlic clove, chopped
- 1 can (15 oz.) white beans, drained
- 1 parsnip, diced
- 1 celery stalk, sliced
- 2 tablespoons Italian pesto
- 1/2 cup chopped parsley
- Salt and pepper to taste

Directions:
1. Combine the chicken, shallot, garlic, beans, parsnip, celery and pesto in a Crock Pot.
2. Add the parsley and season with salt and pepper.
3. Cook on low settings for 6 hours and serve the soup warm and fresh.

Garlicky Spinach Soup With Herbed Croutons

Servings: 6
Cooking Time: 2 1/4 Hours

Ingredients:
- 1 pound fresh spinach, shredded
- 1/2 teaspoon dried oregano
- 1 shallot, chopped
- 4 garlic cloves, chopped
- 1/2 celery stalk, sliced
- 2 cups water
- 2 cups chicken stock
- Salt and pepper to taste
- 1 lemon, juiced
- 1/2 cup half and half
- 10 oz. one-day old bread, cubed
- 3 tablespoons olive oil
- 1 teaspoon dried basil
- 1 teaspoon dried marjoram

Directions:
1. Combine the spinach, oregano, shallot, garlic and

celery in your Crock Pot.
2. Add the water, stock and lemon juice, as well as salt and pepper to taste and cook on high settings for 2 hours.
3. While the soup is cooking, place the bread cubes in a large baking tray and drizzle with olive oil. Sprinkle with salt and pepper and cook in the preheated oven at 375F for 10-12 minutes until crispy and golden.
4. When the soup is done, puree it with an immersion blender, adding the half and half while doing so.
5. Serve the soup warm, topped with herbed croutons.

Crab Stew

Servings:4
Cooking Time: 5 Hours

Ingredients:
- 8 oz crab meat, chopped
- ½ cup mango, chopped
- 1 teaspoon dried lemongrass
- 1 teaspoon ground turmeric
- 1 potato, peeled chopped
- 1 cup of water
- ½ cup of coconut milk

Directions:
1. Put all ingredients in the Crock Pot.
2. Gently stir them with the help of the spoon and close the lid.
3. Cook the stew on low for 5 hours.
4. Then leave the cooked stew for 10-15 minutes to rest.

Nutrition Info:
- Per Serving: 167 calories, 8.9g protein, 13.6g carbohydrates, 8.3g fat, 2.1g fiber, 30mg cholesterol, 364mg sodium, 310mg potassium.

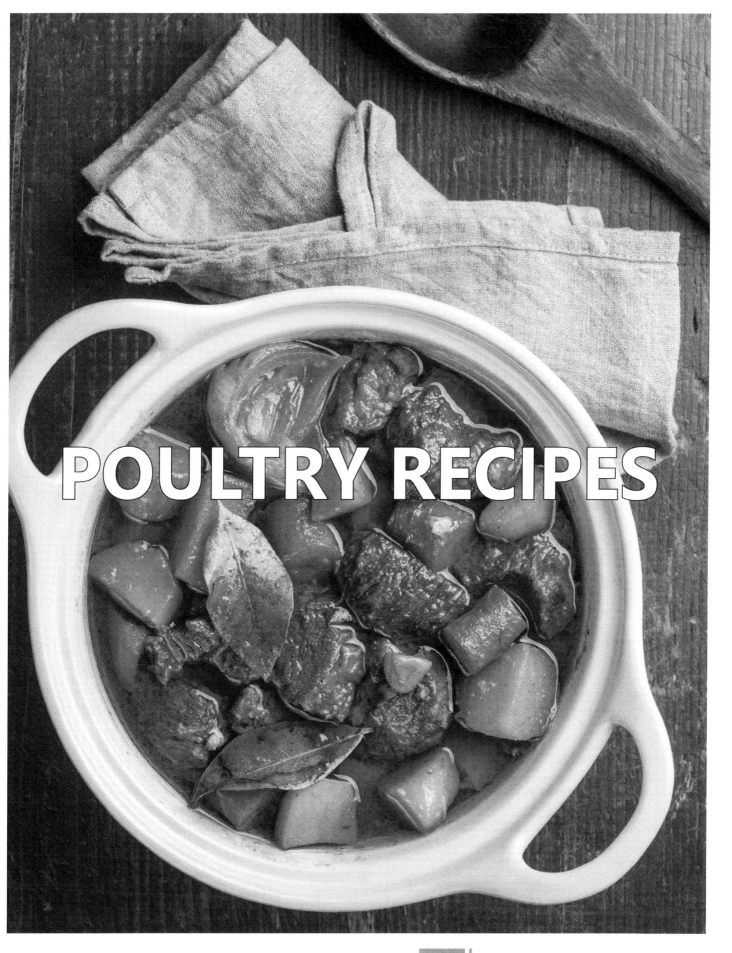

POULTRY RECIPES

Poultry Recipes

Saucy Chicken

Servings: 4
Cooking Time: 5 Hours

Ingredients:
- 1 chicken, cut into medium pieces
- Salt and black pepper to the taste
- 1 tbsp olive oil
- ½ tsp sweet paprika
- ¼ cup white wine
- ½ tsp marjoram, dried
- ¼ cup chicken stock
- 2 tbsp white vinegar
- ¼ cup apricot preserves
- 1 and ½ tsp ginger, grated
- 2 tbsp honey

Directions:
1. Add chicken, marjoram, and all other ingredients to the Crock Pot.
2. Put the cooker's lid on and set the cooking time to 5 hours on Low settings.
3. Serve warm.

Nutrition Info:
- Per Serving: Calories: 230, Total Fat: 3g, Fiber: 5g, Total Carbs: 12g, Protein: 22g

Chicken Thighs And Mushrooms

Servings: 4
Cooking Time: 4 Hours

Ingredients:
- 4 chicken thighs
- 2 cups mushrooms, sliced
- ¼ cup butter, melted
- Salt and black pepper to the taste
- ½ teaspoon onion powder
- ½ teaspoon garlic powder
- ½ cup water
- 1 teaspoon Dijon mustard
- 1 tablespoon tarragon, chopped

Directions:

1. In your Crock Pot, mix chicken with butter, mushrooms, salt, pepper, onion powder, garlic powder, water, mustard and tarragon, toss, cover and cook on High for 4 hours.
2. Divide between plates and serve.

Nutrition Info:
- calories 453, fat 32, fiber 6, carbs 15, protein 36

Chili Sausages

Servings:4
Cooking Time: 3 Hours

Ingredients:
- 1-pound chicken sausages, roughly chopped
- ½ cup of water
- 1 tablespoon chili powder
- 1 teaspoon tomato paste

Directions:
1. Sprinkle the chicken sausages with chili powder and transfer in the Crock Pot.
2. Then mix water and tomato paste and pour the liquid over the chicken sausages.
3. Close the lid and cook the meal on High for 3 hours.

Nutrition Info:
- Per Serving: 221 calories, 15g protein, 8.9g carbohydrates, 12.8g fat, 1.4g fiber, 0mg cholesterol, 475mg sodium, 50mg potassium.

Chicken And Tomatillos

Servings: 6
Cooking Time: 4 Hours

Ingredients:
- 1 pound chicken thighs, skinless and boneless
- 2 tablespoons olive oil
- 1 yellow onion, chopped
- 1 garlic clove, minced
- 4 ounces canned green chilies, chopped
- A handful cilantro, chopped
- Salt and black pepper to the taste

- 15 ounces canned tomatillos, chopped
- 5 ounces canned garbanzo beans, drained
- 15 ounces rice, cooked
- 5 ounces tomatoes, chopped
- 15 ounces cheddar cheese, grated
- 4 ounces black olives, pitted and chopped

Directions:

1. In your Crock Pot, mix oil with onions, garlic, chicken, chilies, salt, pepper, cilantro and tomatillos, stir, cover the Crock Pot and cook on High for 3 hours
2. Take chicken out of the Crock Pot, shred, return to Crock Pot, add rice, beans, cheese, tomatoes and olives, cover and cook on High for 1 more hour.
3. Divide between plates and serve.

Nutrition Info:

- calories 300, fat 11, fiber 3, carbs 14, protein 30

Banana Chicken

Servings:6
Cooking Time: 9 Hours

Ingredients:

- 2 bananas, chopped
- 2-pound whole chicken
- 1 tablespoon taco seasonings
- 1 tablespoon olive oil
- ½ cup of soy sauce
- ½ cup of water

Directions:

1. Fill the chicken with bananas and secure the whole.
2. Then rub the chicken with taco seasonings and brush with olive oil.
3. After this, pour water and soy sauce in the Crock Pot.
4. Add chicken and close the lid.
5. Cook it on Low for 9 hours.

Nutrition Info:

- Per Serving: 360 calories, 45.5g protein, 11.9g carbohydrates, 13.7g fat, 1.2g fiber, 135mg cholesterol, 1469mg sodium, 555mg potassium.

Chicken Piccata

Servings:4
Cooking Time: 8 Hours

Ingredients:

- 4 chicken breasts, skin and bones removed
- Salt and pepper to taste

- ¼ cup butter, cubed
- ¼ cup chicken broth
- 1 tablespoon lemon juice

Directions:

1. Place all ingredients in the crockpot.
2. Give a good stir to combine everything.
3. Close the lid and cook on low for 8 hours or on high for 6 hours.

Nutrition Info:

- Calories per serving: 265; Carbohydrates:2.3 g; Protein:24 g; Fat: 14g; Sugar: 0g; Sodium:442 mg; Fiber:0 g

Crockpot Yellow Chicken Curry

Servings:5
Cooking Time: 8 Hours

Ingredients:

- 1 ½ pounds boneless chicken breasts, cut into chunks
- 6 cups vegetable broth (made from boiling onions, broccoli, bell pepper, and carrots in 7 cups water)
- 1 cup coconut milk, unsweetened
- 1 cup tomatoes, crushed
- 1 tablespoon cumin
- 2 teaspoons ground coriander
- 1 teaspoon turmeric powder
- 1 thumb-size ginger, sliced
- 4 cloves of garlic, minced
- 1 teaspoon cinnamon
- ½ teaspoon cayenne pepper
- Salt to taste

Directions:

1. Place all ingredients in the CrockPot.
2. Close the lid and cook on high for 6 hours or on low for 8 hours.

Nutrition Info:

- Calories per serving: 291; Carbohydrates: 6.1g; Protein: 32.5g; Fat: 15.4g; Sugar: 0.3g; Sodium: 527mg; Fiber: 2.8g

Chicken, Peppers And Onions

Servings:4
Cooking Time: 8 Hours

Ingredients:
- 1 tablespoon olive oil
- ½ cup shallots, peeled
- 1-pound boneless chicken breasts, sliced
- ½ cup green and red peppers, diced
- Salt and pepper to taste

Directions:
1. Heat oil in a skillet over medium flame.
2. Sauté the shallots until fragrant and translucent. Allow to cook so that the outer edges of the shallots turn slightly brown.
3. Transfer into the crockpot.
4. Add the chicken breasts and the peppers.
5. Season with salt and pepper to taste.
6. Add a few tablespoons of water.
7. Close the lid and cook on low for 8 hours or on high for 6 hours.

Nutrition Info:
- Calories per serving: 179; Carbohydrates: 3.05g; Protein:26.1 g; Fat: 10.4g; Sugar: 0g; Sodium: 538mg; Fiber:2.4 g

Mexican Chicken "bake"

Servings:6
Cooking Time: 8 Hours

Ingredients:
- 6 roma tomatoes, cut into quarters
- 1 cup cilantro leaves
- 1 yellow onion, quartered
- 1 teaspoon cumin
- 1 jalapeno, seeded
- 3 cloves of garlic, peeled
- Salt and pepper to taste
- 2 pounds chicken breasts, bones and skin removed
- ½ cup queso quesadilla cheese, shredded
- 1-ounce black olives, pitted and sliced

Directions:
1. Place the tomatoes, cilantro, onion, cumin, jalapeno, and garlic in a food processor. Season with salt and pepper to taste. Pulse until smooth.
2. Place the chicken breasts in the CrockPot and pour over the salsa sauce.
3. Top with cheese and olives.

4. Close the lid and cook on high for 6 hours and on high for 8 hours.
5. Garnish with sour cream, avocado slices, or cilantro.

Nutrition Info:
- Calories per serving: 203; Carbohydrates: 5g; Protein: 18g; Fat: 11g; Sugar: 0g; Sodium:637 mg; Fiber: 1g

Party Chicken Wings

Servings:4
Cooking Time: 4 Hours

Ingredients:
- 1-pound chicken wings
- 3 tablespoons hot sauce
- 2 tablespoons butter
- ¼ cup of soy sauce

Directions:
1. Put all ingredients in the Crock Pot and close the lid.
2. Cook the chicken wings on High for 4 hours.
3. Then transfer the chicken wings in the big bowl and sprinkle with hot sauce gravy from the Crock Pot.

Nutrition Info:
- Per Serving: 276 calories, 33.9g protein, 1.4g carbohydrates, 14.2g fat, 0.2g fiber, 116mg cholesterol, 1322mg sodium, 327mg potassium.

Chicken Parm

Servings:3
Cooking Time: 4 Hours

Ingredients:
- 9 oz chicken fillet
- 1/3 cup cream
- 3 oz Parmesan, grated
- 1 teaspoon olive oil

Directions:
1. Brush the Crock Pot bowl with olive oil from inside.
2. Then slice the chicken fillet and place it in the Crock Pot.
3. Top it with Parmesan and cream.
4. Close the lid and cook the meal on High for 4 hours.

Nutrition Info:
- Per Serving: 283 calories, 33.9g protein, 1.8g car-

bohydrates, 15.4g fat, 0g fiber, 101mg cholesterol, 345mg sodium, 216mg potassium.

Sheriff Chicken Wings

Servings:4
Cooking Time: 3 Hours

Ingredients:
- 1-pound chicken wings
- 1 cup plain yogurt
- ¼ cup pickled cucumbers, grated
- 1 tablespoon lemon juice
- 1 teaspoon white pepper
- 1 teaspoon salt
- 1 teaspoon cayenne pepper
- 1 cup of water

Directions:
1. Put chicken wings in the Crock Pot.
2. Add cayenne pepper and salt.
3. Then add water and cook the chicken on High for 3 hours.
4. Meanwhile, mix plain yogurt with grated pickled cucumbers, and white pepper.
5. When the chicken wings are cooked, transfer them in the serving plates and top with plain yogurt sauce.

Nutrition Info:
• Per Serving: 264 calories, 36.5g protein, 5.2g carbohydrates, 9.3g fat, 0.3g fiber, 105mg cholesterol, 725mg sodium, 450mg potassium.

Honey Turkey Breast

Servings:4
Cooking Time: 3.5 Hours

Ingredients:
- 1-pound turkey breast, skinless, boneless
- 3 tablespoons of liquid honey
- 1 teaspoon chili powder
- 1 teaspoon smoked paprika
- ½ teaspoon salt
- 1 cup of water
- 3 tablespoons butter

Directions:
1. Sprinkle the turkey breast with salt, smoked paprika, and chili powder.
2. Put the turkey in the Crock Pot, add water, and close the lid.
3. Cook the meal on High for 3 hours.

4. Then drain water and sprinkle the turkey breast with butter and liquid honey. Carefully mix the turkey breast and cook it on High for 30 minutes.

Nutrition Info:
• Per Serving: 246 calories, 19.7g protein, 18.4g carbohydrates, 10.7g fat, 1g fiber, 72mg cholesterol, 1512mg sodium, 379mg potassium.

Wine Chicken

Servings:4
Cooking Time: 3 Hours

Ingredients:
- 1 cup red wine
- 1-pound chicken breast, skinless, boneless, chopped
- 1 anise star
- 1 teaspoon cayenne pepper
- 2 garlic cloves, crushed

Directions:
1. Pour red wine in the Crock Pot.
2. Add anise star, cayenne pepper, and garlic cloves.
3. Then add chopped chicken and close the lid.
4. Cook the meal on High for 3 hours.
5. Serve the chicken with hot wine sauce.

Nutrition Info:
• Per Serving: 182 calories, 24.2g protein, 2.4g carbohydrates, 2.9g fat, 0.2g fiber, 73mg cholesterol, 61mg sodium, 493mg potassium.

Bbq Chicken

Servings:2
Cooking Time: 7 Hours

Ingredients:
- 1 teaspoon minced garlic
- ½ cup BBQ sauce
- 1 tablespoon avocado oil
- 3 tablespoons lemon juice
- ½ cup of water
- 7 oz chicken fillet, sliced

Directions:
1. In the bowl BBQ sauce, minced garlic, avocado oil, and lemon juice.
2. Add chicken fillet and mix the mixture.
3. After this, transfer it to the Crock Pot. Add water and close the lid.
4. Cook the chicken on low for 7 hours.

Nutrition Info:

- Per Serving: 299 calories, 29.1g protein, 24g carbohydrates, 8.6g fat, 0.8g fiber, 88mg cholesterol, 792mg sodium, 428mg potassium.

Duck Chili

Servings: 4
Cooking Time: 7

Ingredients:
- 1 pound northern beans, soaked and rinsed
- 1 yellow onion, cut into half
- 1 garlic heat, top trimmed off
- Salt and black pepper to the taste
- 2 cloves
- 1 bay leaf
- 6 cups water
- For the duck:
- 1 pound duck, ground
- 1 tablespoon vegetable oil
- 1 yellow onion, minced
- 2 carrots, chopped
- Salt and black pepper to the taste
- 4 ounces canned green chilies and their juice
- 1 teaspoon brown sugar
- 15 ounces canned tomatoes and their juices, chopped
- A handful cilantro, chopped

Directions:
1. Put the beans in your Crock Pot, add the whole onion, garlic head, cloves, bay leaf, the water and salt to the taste, stir, cover, cook on High for 4 hours, drain them and put them in a bowl.
2. Clean the Crock Pot, add oil, carrots, chopped onion, season with salt and pepper, duck, chilies, tomatoes and sugar, stir, cover and cook on High for 3 hours more.
3. Divide on duck and beans mix plates and serve with cilantro sprinkled on top.

Nutrition Info:
- calories 283, fat 15, fiber 2, carbs 16, protein 22

Citrus Glazed Chicken

Servings: 4
Cooking Time: 4 Hrs

Ingredients:
- 2 lbs. chicken thighs, skinless, boneless and cut into pieces
- Salt and black pepper to the taste
- 3 tbsp olive oil

- ¼ cup flour
- For the sauce:
- 2 tbsp fish sauce
- 1 and ½ tsp orange extract
- 1 tbsp ginger, grated
- ¼ cup of orange juice
- 2 tsp sugar
- 1 tbsp orange zest
- ¼ tsp sesame seeds
- 2 tbsp scallions, chopped
- ½ tsp coriander, ground
- 1 cup of water
- ¼ tsp red pepper flakes
- 2 tbsp soy sauce

Directions:
1. Whisk flour with black pepper, salt, and chicken pieces in a bowl to coat well.
2. Add chicken to a pan greased with oil and sear it over medium heat until golden brown.
3. Transfer the chicken to the Crock Pot.
4. Blend orange juice, fish sauce, soy sauce, ginger, water, coriander, orange extract, and stevia in a blender jug.
5. Pour this fish sauce mixture over the chicken and top it with orange zest, scallions, sesame seeds, and pepper flakes.
6. Put the cooker's lid on and set the cooking time to 4 hours on High settings.
7. Serve warm.

Nutrition Info:
- Per Serving: Calories: 423, Total Fat: 20g, Fiber: 5g, Total Carbs: 12g, Protein: 45g

Chicken And Olives

Servings: 2
Cooking Time: 5 Hours

Ingredients:
- 1 pound chicken breasts, skinless, boneless and sliced
- 1 cup black olives, pitted and halved
- ½ cup chicken stock
- ½ cup tomato sauce
- 1 tablespoon lime juice
- 1 tablespoon lime zest, grated
- 1 teaspoon chili powder
- 2 spring onions, chopped
- 1 tablespoon chives, chopped

Directions:
1. In your Crock Pot, mix the chicken with the olives, stock and the other ingredients except the chives, toss, put the lid on and cook on High for 5 hours.
2. Divide the mix into bowls, sprinkle the chives on top and serve.

Nutrition Info:
- calories 200, fat 7, fiber 1, carbs 5, protein 12

Tomato Chicken And Chickpeas

Servings: 2
Cooking Time: 7 Hours

Ingredients:
- 1 tablespoon olive oil
- 1 red onion, chopped
- 1 cup canned chickpeas, drained
- 1 pound chicken breast, skinless, boneless and cubed
- ½ cup tomato sauce
- ½ cup cherry tomatoes, halved
- ½ teaspoon rosemary, dried
- ½ teaspoon turmeric powder
- 1 cup chicken stock
- A pinch of salt and black pepper
- 1 tablespoon chives, chopped

Directions:
1. Grease the Crock Pot with the oil and mix the chicken with the onion, chickpeas and the other ingredients inside the pot.
2. Put the lid on, cook on Low for 7 hours, divide between plates and serve.

Nutrition Info:
- calories 291, fat 17, fiber 3, carbs 7, protein 16

Salsa Chicken Wings

Servings:5
Cooking Time: 6 Hours

Ingredients:
- 2-pounds chicken wings
- 2 cups salsa
- ½ cup of water

Directions:
1. Put all ingredients in the Crock Pot.
2. Carefully mix the mixture and close the lid.
3. Cook the chicken wings on low for 6 hours.

Nutrition Info:

- Per Serving: 373 calories, 54.1g protein, 6.5g carbohydrates, 13.6g fat, 1.7g fiber, 161mg cholesterol, 781mg sodium, 750mg potassium.

Chicken Chickpeas

Servings: 4
Cooking Time: 4 Hrs

Ingredients:
- 1 yellow onion, chopped
- 2 tbsp butter
- 4 garlic cloves, minced
- 1 tbsp ginger, grated
- 1 and ½ tsp paprika
- 1 tbsp cumin, ground
- 1 and ½ tsp coriander, ground
- 1 tsp turmeric, ground
- Salt and black pepper to the taste
- A pinch of cayenne pepper
- 15 oz. canned tomatoes, crushed
- ¼ cup lemon juice
- 1 lb. spinach, chopped
- 3 lbs. chicken drumsticks and thighs
- ½ cup cilantro, chopped
- ½ cup chicken stock
- 15 oz. canned chickpeas, drained
- ½ cup heavy cream

Directions:
1. Grease the base of the Crock Pot with butter.
2. Stir in chicken, chickpeas, and all other ingredients to the Crock Pot.
3. Put the cooker's lid on and set the cooking time to 4 hours on High settings.
4. Serve warm.

Nutrition Info:
- Per Serving: Calories: 300, Total Fat: 4g, Fiber: 6g, Total Carbs: 30g, Protein: 17g

Halved Chicken

Servings:4
Cooking Time: 5 Hours

Ingredients:
- 2-pounds whole chicken, halved
- 1 tablespoon salt
- 1 teaspoon ground black pepper
- 2 tablespoons mayonnaise
- ½ cup of water

Directions:
1. Mix the ground black pepper with salt and mayonnaise.
2. Then rub the chicken halves with mayonnaise mixture and transfer in the Crock Pot.
3. Add water and close the lid.
4. Cook the chicken on High for 5 hours.

Nutrition Info:
- Per Serving: 461 calories, 65.7g protein, 2.1g carbohydrates, 19.3g fat, 1.2g fiber, 0.1mg cholesterol, 1993mg sodium, 559mg potassium.

Chicken With Mushroom Sauce

Servings: 4
Cooking Time: 4 Hrs

Ingredients:
- 8 chicken thighs
- Salt and black pepper to the taste
- 1 yellow onion, chopped
- 1 tbsp olive oil
- 4 bacon strips, cooked and chopped
- 4 garlic cloves, minced
- 10 oz. cremini mushrooms halved
- 2 cups white chardonnay wine
- 1 cup whipping cream
- Handful parsley, chopped

Directions:
1. Add oil, chicken pieces, black pepper, and salt to a pan.
2. Stir cook the chicken until it turns golden brown.
3. Transfer the chicken to the Crock Pot and the remaining ingredients.
4. Put the cooker's lid on and set the cooking time to 4 hours on High settings.
5. Serve warm.

Nutrition Info:
- Per Serving: Calories: 340, Total Fat: 10g, Fiber:

7g, Total Carbs: 14g, Protein: 24g

Chicken Provolone

Servings:4
Cooking Time: 8 Hours

Ingredients:
- 4 chicken breasts, bones and skin removed
- Salt and pepper to taste
- 8 fresh basil leaves
- 4 slices prosciutto
- 4 slices provolone cheese

Directions:
1. Sprinkle the chicken breasts with salt and pepper to taste.
2. Place in the crockpot and add the basil leaves, and prosciutto on top.
3. Arrange the provolone cheese slices on top.
4. Close the lid and cook on low for 8 hours and on high for 6 hours.

Nutrition Info:
- Calories per serving: 236; Carbohydrates: 1g; Protein: 33g; Fat: 11g; Sugar:0 g; Sodium: 435mg; Fiber:0 g

Chicken Masala

Servings:4
Cooking Time: 4 Hours

Ingredients:
- 1 teaspoon garam masala
- 1 teaspoon ground ginger
- 1 cup of coconut milk
- 1-pound chicken fillet, sliced
- 1 teaspoon olive oil

Directions:
1. Mix coconut milk with ground ginger, garam masala, and olive oil.
2. Add chicken fillet and mix the ingredients.
3. Then transfer them in the Crock Pot and cook on High for 4 hours.

Nutrition Info:
- Per Serving: 365 calories, 34.2g protein, 3.6g carbohydrates, 23.9g fat, 1.4g fiber, 101mg cholesterol, 108mg sodium, 439mg potassium.

Coconut Turmeric Chicken

Servings: 8
Cooking Time: 8 Hours

Ingredients:
- 1 whole chicken, cut into pieces
- ½ cup coconut milk, unsweetened
- 2 inch-knob fresh turmeric, grated
- 2 inch-knob fresh ginger, grated
- 4 cloves of garlic, grated
- Salt and pepper to taste

Directions:
1. Place all ingredients in the CrockPot.
2. Close the lid and cook on high for 6 hours or on low for 8 hours.
3. Garnish with chopped scallions.

Nutrition Info:
- Calories per serving: 270; Carbohydrates: 4.2g; Protein:24.5g; Fat: 18.9g; Sugar: 0g; Sodium: 883mg; Fiber: 1.6g

Turkey Soup With Rosemary And Kale

Servings: 6
Cooking Time: 8 Hours

Ingredients:
- ½ onion, chopped
- 2 cloves of garlic, minced
- Salt and pepper to taste
- 1 tablespoon tallow or ghee
- 1-pound turkey meat, cut into bite-sized pieces
- 4 cups homemade chicken stock
- 2 sprigs rosemary, chopped
- 3 cups kale, chopped

Directions:
1. Place all ingredients except the kale in the Crock-Pot.
2. Close the lid and cook on high for 6 hours or on low for 8 hours.
3. An hour before the cooking time ends, add in the kale.
4. Close the lid and cook until the kale has wilted.

Nutrition Info:
- Calories per serving: 867; Carbohydrates: 2.6g; Protein: 151.3g; Fat: 23.6g; Sugar: 0g; Sodium: 1373mg; Fiber: 1.4g

Curry Drumsticks

Servings: 4
Cooking Time: 3 Hours

Ingredients:
- 8 chicken drumsticks
- 1 cup cream
- 1 teaspoon curry paste
- 1 teaspoon olive oil

Directions:
1. Mix the curry paste with cream and pour the liquid in the Crock Pot.
2. Add olive oil and chicken drumsticks.
3. Close the lid and cook the chicken on High for 3 hours.

Nutrition Info:
- Per Serving: 212 calories, 25.8g protein, 2.2g carbohydrates, 10.5g fat, 0g fiber, 92mg cholesterol, 93mg sodium, 205mg potassium.

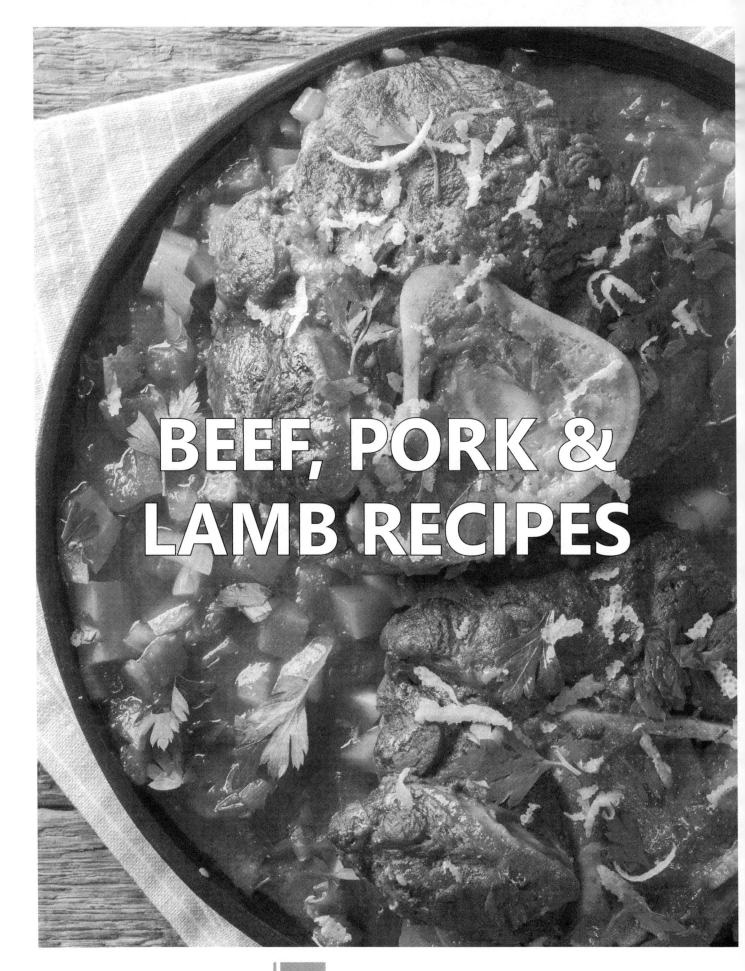

BEEF, PORK & LAMB RECIPES

Sautéed Beef Liver

Servings:4
Cooking Time: 5 Hours

Ingredients:

- 12 oz beef liver, cut into strips
- 1 cup of water
- ½ cup cream
- 1 teaspoon salt
- 1 teaspoon ground black pepper
- 1 onion, sliced
- 1 tablespoon flour
- 1 tablespoon butter

Directions:

1. Sprinkle the beef liver with ground black pepper and salt.
2. Then sprinkle it with flour.
3. After this, put the sliced onion in the Crock Pot in one layer.
4. Add the layer of the liver.
5. Then add water, butter, and cream.
6. Close the lid and cook the meal on high for 5 hours.

Nutrition Info:

- Per Serving: 213 calories, 23.4g protein, 9.7g carbohydrates, 8.6g fat, 0.8g fiber, 337mg cholesterol, 680mg sodium, 360mg potassium.

Honey Pork Chops

Servings: 2
Cooking Time: 5 Hours

Ingredients:

- 2 teaspoons avocado oil
- 1 pound pork chops, bone in
- 2 tablespoons mayonnaise
- 1 tablespoon ketchup
- ½ tablespoon honey
- ¼ cup beef stock
- ½ tablespoon lime juice

Directions:

1. In your Crock Pot, mix the pork chops with the oil, honey and the other ingredients, toss well, put the lid on, and cook on High for 5 hours.
2. Divide pork chops between plates and serve.

Nutrition Info:

- calories 300, fat 8, fiber 10, carbs 16, protein 16

Cauliflower And Beef Ragout

Servings:4
Cooking Time: 4 Hours

Ingredients:

- 2 cups cauliflower florets, chopped
- 2 tablespoons tomato paste
- 1 onion, sliced
- 1 teaspoon ground black pepper
- 2 cups of water
- 7 oz beef loin, chopped
- 1 tablespoon avocado oil

Directions:

1. Mix the beef loin with ground black pepper and put it in the skillet.
2. Add avocado oil and roast the beef for 3 minutes per side.
3. Transfer the meat in the Crock Pot.
4. Add all remaining ingredients and close the lid.
5. Cook the ragout on High for 4 hours.

Nutrition Info:

- Per Serving: 110 calories, 10.9g protein, 7.9g carbohydrates, 4.1g fat, 2.5g fiber, 27mg cholesterol, 246mg sodium, 292mg potassium.

Beef Meatballs Casserole

Servings: 8
Cooking Time: 7 Hours

Ingredients:
- 1/3 cup flour
- 2 eggs
- 1 pound beef sausage, chopped
- 1 pound beef, ground
- Salt and black pepper to taste
- 1 tablespoons parsley, dried
- ¼ teaspoon red pepper flakes
- ¼ cup parmesan, grated
- ¼ teaspoon onion powder
- ½ teaspoon garlic powder
- ¼ teaspoon oregano, dried
- 1 cup ricotta cheese
- 2 cups marinara sauce
- 1 and ½ cups mozzarella cheese, shredded

Directions:
1. In a bowl, mix sausage with beef, salt, pepper, almond flour, parsley, pepper flakes, onion powder, garlic powder, oregano, parmesan and eggs, stir well and shape meatballs out of this mix.
2. Arrange meatballs in your Crock Pot, add half of the marinara sauce, ricotta cheese and top with the rest of the marinara.
3. Add mozzarella at the end, cover and cook on Low for 7 hours.
4. Divide between plates and serve.

Nutrition Info:
- calories 456, fat 35, fiber 3, carbs 12, protein 32

Beef Bolognese

Servings:4
Cooking Time: 5 Hours

Ingredients:
- ½ cup onion, diced
- 1 teaspoon dried basil
- 1 teaspoon dried cilantro
- ½ cup tomato juice
- 1 tablespoon sesame oil
- 1-pound ground beef
- 2 oz parmesan, grated

Directions:
1. In the mixing bowl mix ground beef with cilantro, basil, and onion.

2. Pour the sesame oil in the Crock Pot.
3. Add tomato juice and ground beef mixture.
4. Cook it on high for 3 hours.
5. Then add parmesan and carefully mix.
6. Cook the meal on low for 2 hours more.

Nutrition Info:
- Per Serving: 297 calories, 39.4g protein, 3.2g carbohydrates, 13.5g fat, 0.4g fiber, 111mg cholesterol, 289mg sodium, 548mg potassium.

Sweet And Sour Pulled Pork

Servings:4
Cooking Time: 6 Hours

Ingredients:
- 1-pound pork sirloin
- 2 cups of water
- 2 tablespoons ketchup
- 2 tablespoons lemon juice
- 1 teaspoon cayenne pepper
- 1 teaspoon liquid honey

Directions:
1. Pour water in the Crock Pot.
2. Add pork sirloin and close the lid.
3. Cook the meat on high for 6 hours.
4. Then drain water and shred the meat.
5. Add ketchup, lemon juice, cayenne pepper, and liquid honey.
6. Stir the mixture carefully and transfer in the serving plates.

Nutrition Info:
- Per Serving: 207 calories, 23.3g protein, 3.7g carbohydrates, 10.2g fat, 0.2g fiber, 80mg cholesterol, 154mg sodium, 49mg potassium.

Lamb Saute

Servings:5
Cooking Time: 4.5 Hours

Ingredients:
- 1 cup tomatoes, chopped
- 1 cup bell pepper, chopped
- 1 chili pepper, chopped
- 1 tablespoon avocado oil
- 12 oz lamb fillet, chopped
- ½ cup cremini mushrooms, sliced
- 1 cup of water

Directions:

1. Heat the avocado oil in the skillet well.
2. Add chopped lamb and roast it for 5 minutes. Stir the meat from time to time.
3. After this, transfer the meat in the Crock Pot and add all remaining ingredients.
4. Close the lid and cook the saute on High for 5 hours.

Nutrition Info:
• Per Serving: 147 calories, 19.9g protein, 3.7g carbohydrates, 5.5g fat, 0.9g fiber, 61mg cholesterol, 56mg sodium, 402mg potassium.

Pork Sirloin Salsa Mix

Servings: 4
Cooking Time: 8 Hours

Ingredients:
• 2 pounds pork sirloin roast, cut into thick slices
• Salt and black pepper to the taste
• 2 teaspoons garlic powder
• 2 teaspoons cumin, ground
• 1 tablespoon olive oil
• 16 ounces green chili tomatillo salsa

Directions:
1. In your Crock Pot, mix pork with cumin, salt, pepper and garlic powder and rub well.
2. Add oil and salsa, toss, cover and cook on Low for 8 hours.
3. Divide between plates and serve hot.

Nutrition Info:
• calories 400, fat 7, fiber 6, carbs 10, protein 25

Mustard Beef

Servings:4
Cooking Time: 8 Hours

Ingredients:
• 1-pound beef sirloin, chopped
• 1 tablespoon capers, drained
• 1 cup of water
• 2 tablespoons mustard
• 1 tablespoon coconut oil

Directions:
1. Mix meat with mustard and leave for 10 minutes to marinate.
2. Then melt the coconut oil in the skillet.
3. Add meat and roast it for 1 minute per side on high heat.

4. After this, transfer the meat in the Crock Pot.
5. Add water and capers.
6. Cook the meal on Low for 8 hours.

Nutrition Info:
• Per Serving: 267 calories, 35.9g protein, 2.1g carbohydrates, 12.1g fat, 0.9g fiber, 101mg cholesterol, 140mg sodium, 496mg potassium.

Beef Heart In Creamy Gravy

Servings:4
Cooking Time: 6 Hours

Ingredients:
• 12 oz beef heart, cut into slices
• 1 cup cream
• 1 teaspoon cornflour
• 1 teaspoon salt
• 3 garlic cloves, diced
• 1 tablespoon butter

Directions:
1. Sprinkle the beef heart with salt and cornflour.
2. Then put butter in the Crock Pot.
3. Add a beef heart, garlic, and cream.
4. Close the lid and cook the meal on Low for 6 hours.

Nutrition Info:
• Per Serving: 210 calories, 24.9g protein, 3.2g carbohydrates, 10.3g fat, 0.1g fiber, 199mg cholesterol, 672mg sodium, 220mg potassium.

Beef Sausages In Maple Syrup

Servings:4
Cooking Time: 5 Hours

Ingredients:
• 1-pound beef sausages
• ½ cup maple syrup
• 3 tablespoons butter
• 1 teaspoon ground cumin
• ¼ cup of water

Directions:
1. Toss butter in the skillet and melt it.
2. Then pour the melted butter in the Crock Pot.
3. Add water, cumin, and maple syrup. Stir the liquid until smooth.
4. Add beef sausages and close the lid.
5. Cook the meal on High for 5 hours.

Nutrition Info:
• Per Serving: 630 calories, 15.8 g protein, 29.7g

carbohydrates, 50g fat, 0.1g fiber, 103mg cholesterol, 979mg sodium, 307mg potassium.

Lamb And Kale

Servings: 2
Cooking Time: 4 Hours

Ingredients:
- 1 pound lamb shoulder, cubed
- 1 cup baby kale
- 1 tablespoon olive oil
- 1 yellow onion, chopped
- ½ teaspoon coriander, ground
- ½ teaspoon cumin, ground
- ½ teaspoon sweet paprika
- A pinch of salt and black pepper
- ¼ cup beef stock
- 1 tablespoon chives, chopped

Directions:
1. In your Crock Pot, mix the lamb with the kale, oil, onion and the other ingredients, toss, put the lid on and cook on High for 4 hours.
2. Divide everything between plates and serve.

Nutrition Info:
- calories 264, fat 14, fiber 3, carbs 6, protein 17

Pork Sweet Potato Stew

Servings: 6
Cooking Time: 4 Hrs.

Ingredients:
- 1 lb. sweet potatoes, chopped
- 3 and ½ lbs. pork roast
- 8 medium carrots, chopped
- Salt and black pepper to the taste
- 15 oz. canned tomatoes, chopped
- 1 yellow onion, chopped
- Grated zest and juice of 1 lemon
- 4 garlic cloves, minced
- 3 bay leaves
- Black pepper to the taste
- ½ cup kalamata olives pitted

Directions:
1. Add potatoes, carrots, and all other ingredients except the olives to the insert of the Crock Pot.
2. Put the cooker's lid on and set the cooking time to 4 hours on High settings.
3. Discard the bay leaves and transfer the meat to the serving plate.
4. Roughly mash the remaining veggies and add olives.
5. Transfer the veggies mix to the serving plate.
6. Serve warm.

Nutrition Info:
- Per Serving: Calories: 250, Total Fat: 4g, Fiber: 3g, Total Carbs: 6g, Protein: 13g

Beef San Marco Steak

Servings:4
Cooking Time: 5 Hours

Ingredients:
- 4 beef steaks
- 2 tablespoons avocado oil
- 1 teaspoon minced garlic
- 1 teaspoon dried oregano
- 1 tablespoon balsamic vinegar
- ½ cup onion soup, canned
- ¼ cup red wine

Directions:
1. Rub the beef steaks with minced ginger, dried oregano, and sprinkle with balsamic vinegar.
2. Transfer the beef steaks in the Crock Pot.
3. Add all remaining ingredients from the list above and close the lid.
4. Cook the meal on High for 5 hours.

Nutrition Info:
- Per Serving: 197 calories, 26.9g protein, 3.3g carbohydrates, 6.7g fat, 0.7g fiber, 76mg cholesterol, 322mg sodium, 409mg potassium.

Lamb Semolina Meatballs

Servings: 6
Cooking Time: 5 Hrs.

Ingredients:
- 1 red onion, peeled and grated
- 1 tbsp semolina
- 2 tbsp dried parsley
- 1 tsp chili flakes
- 1 tsp ground black pepper
- 1 tsp oregano
- 1 lb. minced lamb
- 2 tbsp minced garlic
- 1 tsp onion powder
- 1 tbsp butter

- 1 egg

Directions:

1. Mix minced lamb with onion, parsley, chili flakes, black pepper, onion powder, minced garlic, oregano, and semolina in a bowl.
2. Add egg and mix the minced meat mixture with the help of your hands.
3. Make small meatballs of this lamb mixture and keep them aside.
4. Add melted butter along with the meatballs to the insert of the Crock Pot.
5. Put the cooker's lid on and set the cooking time to 3 hours on High settings.
6. Serve warm.

Nutrition Info:
- Per Serving: Calories: 256, Total Fat: 16.4g, Fiber: 1g, Total Carbs: 5.53g, Protein: 21g

5-ingredients Chili

Servings:4
Cooking Time: 5 Hours

Ingredients:
- 8 oz ground beef
- ½ cup Cheddar cheese, shredded
- 2 cup tomatoes, chopped
- 1 teaspoon chili seasonings
- ½ cup of water

Directions:

1. Mix the ground beef with chili seasonings and transfer in the Crock Pot.
2. Add tomatoes and water.
3. Close the lid and cook the chili on high for 3 hours.
4. After this, open the lid and mix the chili well. Top it with cheddar cheese and close the lid.
5. Cook the chili on low for 2 hours more.

Nutrition Info:
- Per Serving: 180 calories, 21.6g protein, 4g carbohydrates, 8.4g fat, 1.1g fiber, 66mg cholesterol, 150mg sodium, 456mg potassium.

Aromatic Lamb

Servings:4
Cooking Time: Hours

Ingredients:
- 1 tablespoon minced garlic
- 1 teaspoon ground black pepper
- ½ teaspoon salt
- 1 teaspoon sesame oil
- 1-pound lamb sirloin, chopped
- ½ cup of water

Directions:

1. Mix the lamb with minced garlic, ground black pepper, and salt.
2. Then sprinkle the meat with sesame oil and transfer in the Crock Pot.
3. Add water and cook the meat on low for 8 hours.

Nutrition Info:
- Per Serving: 246 calories, 32.3g protein, 1g carbohydrates, 11.6g fat, 0.2g fiber, 104mg cholesterol, 373mg sodium, 393mg potassium.

Pork Rolls

Servings:2
Cooking Time: 4.5 Hours

Ingredients:
- 2 pork chops
- 2 oz Mozzarella, sliced
- 1 teaspoon cayenne pepper
- ¼ teaspoon salt
- 1 tablespoon mayonnaise
- ½ cup of water

Directions:

1. Beat the pork chops gently and sprinkle with cayenne pepper and salt.
2. Then brush one side of pork chops with mayonnaise and top with mozzarella.
3. Roll the pork chops and secure the prepared rolls with toothpicks.
4. Place the pork rolls in the Crock Pot.
5. Add water and cook them on High for 4.5 hours.

Nutrition Info:
- Per Serving: 308 calories, 15.1g protein, 19.8g carbohydrates, 18.7g fat, 1.9g fiber, 30mg cholesterol, 1103mg sodium, 19mg potassium

Bavarian Style Sausages

Servings:4
Cooking Time: 4 Hours

Ingredients:
- 12 oz beef sausages
- ½ cup beer
- ¼ cup tomato sauce
- 1 tablespoon garlic, crushed
- 1 tablespoon olive oil
- 1 teaspoon cumin seeds

Directions:
1. In the mixing bowl, mix olive oil with cumin seeds, crushed garlic, and tomato sauce.
2. Then sprinkle the beef sausages with olive oil mixture and put in the Crock Pot.
3. Add tomato sauce and beer.
4. Close the lid and cook the meal on high for 4 hours.

Nutrition Info:
- Per Serving: 361 calories, 12.3g protein, 5.2g carbohydrates, 31.2g fat, 0.4g fiber, 60mg cholesterol, 786mg sodium, 238mg potassium.

Hamburger Style Stuffing

Servings:4
Cooking Time: 3 Hours

Ingredients:
- 1-pound ground pork
- ½ cup Cheddar cheese, shredded
- ½ cup fresh cilantro, chopped
- ¼ cup onion, minced
- 1 cup of water
- ¼ cup tomato juice
- 1 bell pepper, diced
- 1 teaspoon salt

Directions:
1. Mix ground pork with cilantro, onion, and diced pepper.
2. Then transfer the mixture in the Crock Pot.
3. Add all remaining ingredients and mix.
4. Close the lid and cook the stuffing on High for 3 hours.

Nutrition Info:
- Per Serving: 235 calories, 33.7g protein, 3.8g carbohydrates, 8.8g fat, 0.7g fiber, 98mg cholesterol, 778mg sodium, 604mg potassium

Creamy Lamb

Servings: 2
Cooking Time: 6 Hours

Ingredients:
- 2 pounds lamb shoulder, cubed
- 1 cup heavy cream
- 1/3 cup beef stock
- 2 teaspoons avocado oil
- 1 teaspoon turmeric powder
- 1 red onion, sliced
- A pinch of salt and black pepper
- 1 tablespoon cilantro, chopped

Directions:
1. In your Crock Pot, mix the lamb with the stock, oil and the other ingredients except the cream, toss, put the lid on and cook on Low for 5 hours.
2. Add the cream, toss, cook on Low for 1 more hour, divide the mix into bowls and serve.

Nutrition Info:
- calories 233, fat 7, fiber 2, carbs 6, protein 12

Delightful Pepperoncini Beef

Servings:4
Cooking Time: 5 Hours

Ingredients:
- 2 oz pepperoncini
- 1-pound beef chuck roast
- 2 cups of water
- 1 teaspoon minced garlic

Directions:
1. Chop the beef roughly and mix with minced garlic.
2. Then transfer the beef in the Crock Pot.
3. Add water and pepperoncini.
4. Close the lid and cook the meal on High for 5 hours.

Nutrition Info:
- Per Serving: 418 calories, 29.9g protein, 1.7g carbohydrates, 31.6g fat, 0g fiber, 117mg cholesterol, 216mg sodium, 263mg potassium.

Oregano Pork Strips

Servings: 4
Cooking Time: 7 Hours

Ingredients:
- 12 oz pork tenderloin, cut into strips
- 1 tablespoon dried oregano
- 1 cup of water
- 1 teaspoon salt

Directions:
1. Place pork strips in the Crock Pot.
2. Add all remaining ingredients and close the lid.
3. Cook the pork strips on Low for 7 hours.
4. Serve the cooked meal with hot gravy from the Crock Pot.

Nutrition Info:
- Per Serving: 125 calories, 22.4g protein, 0.7g carbohydrates, 3.1g fat, 0.5g fiber, 62mg cholesterol, 632mg sodium, 378mg potassium

Pork Chops And Pineapple Mix

Servings: 4
Cooking Time: 6 Hours

Ingredients:
- 2 pounds pork chops
- 1/3 cup sugar
- ¼ cup ketchup
- 15 ounces pineapple, cubed
- 3 tablespoons apple cider vinegar
- 5 tablespoons soy sauce
- 2 teaspoons garlic, minced
- 3 tablespoons flour

Directions:
1. In a bowl, mix ketchup with sugar, vinegar, soy sauce and tapioca, whisk well, add pork chops, toss well and transfer everything to your Crock Pot
2. Add pineapple and garlic, toss again, cover, cook on Low for 6 hours, divide everything between plates and serve.

Nutrition Info:
- calories 345, fat 5, fiber 6, carbs 13, protein 14

Italian Sausage Soup

Servings: 12
Cooking Time: 6 Hours

Ingredients:
- 64 ounces chicken stock
- 1 teaspoon olive oil
- 1 cup heavy cream
- 10 ounces spinach
- 6 bacon slices, chopped
- 1 pound radishes, chopped
- 2 garlic cloves, minced
- Salt and black pepper to the taste
- A pinch of red pepper flakes, crushed
- 1 yellow onion, chopped
- 1 and ½ pounds hot pork sausage, chopped

Directions:
1. Heat up a pan with the oil over medium-high heat, add sausage, onion and garlic, stir, brown for a few minutes and transfer to your Crock Pot.
2. Add stock, spinach, radishes, bacon, cream, salt, pepper and red pepper flakes, stir, cover and cook on Low for 6 hours.
3. Ladle soup into bowls and serve.

Nutrition Info:
- calories 291, fat 22, fiber 2, carbs 14, protein 17

Italian Pork Roast

Servings: 10
Cooking Time: 12 Hours

Ingredients:
- 5 pounds pork shoulder, bone in
- 7 cloves of garlic, slivered
- 1 tablespoon salt
- 1 teaspoon dried oregano
- 1 teaspoon dried basil
- 1 teaspoon dried rosemary
- ½ teaspoon black pepper

Directions:
1. Place all ingredients in the CrockPot.
2. Give a good stir.
3. Close the lid and cook on high for 10 hours or on low for 12 hours.

Nutrition Info:
- Calories per serving:610; Carbohydrates: 0.9g; Protein: 57.1g; Fat: 40.8g; Sugar: 0g; Sodium: 1240mg; Fiber: 0.2g

Cumin Pork

Servings: 6
Cooking Time: 5 Hours

Ingredients:
- 1-pound pork shoulder, chopped
- 1 teaspoon cumin seeds
- 1 teaspoon garlic powder
- 1 teaspoon ground nutmeg
- 1 carrot, diced
- 2 cup of water
- 1 teaspoon salt

Directions:
1. Roast the cumin seeds in the skillet for 2-3 minutes or until the seeds start to smell.
2. Then place them in the Crock Pot.
3. Add all remaining ingredients and close the lid.
4. Cook the pork on high for 5 hours.

Nutrition Info:
- Per Serving: 230 calories, 17.8g protein, 1.7g carbohydrates, 16.4g fat, 0.4g fiber, 68mg cholesterol, 449mg sodium, 295mg potassium

Ground Beef Zucchini Squares

Servings: 4
Cooking Time: 4.5 Hours

Ingredients:
- 2 large zucchinis, trimmed
- 2 tablespoons ricotta cheese
- 9 oz ground beef
- 1 teaspoon ground black pepper
- ½ cup of water
- 1 teaspoon butter

Directions:
1. Slice the zucchini into strips.
2. Then put butter in the Crock Pot and melt it.
3. Add ground beef and ground black pepper.
4. Roast the meat mixture for 5 minutes.
5. After this, add ricotta cheese and carefully mix.
6. Make the cross from 2 zucchini strips.
7. Put the small amount of the ground beef mixture in the center of the zucchini cross and wrap it into squares.
8. Repeat the same steps with all remaining zucchini and meat mixture.
9. Put the zucchini squares in the Crock Pot.
10. Add water and close the lid.
11. Cook the meal on High for 4.5 hours.

Nutrition Info:
- Per Serving: 165 calories, 22.3g protein, 6.2g carbohydrates, 5.9g fat, 1.9g fiber, 62mg cholesterol, 76mg sodium, 697mg potassium.

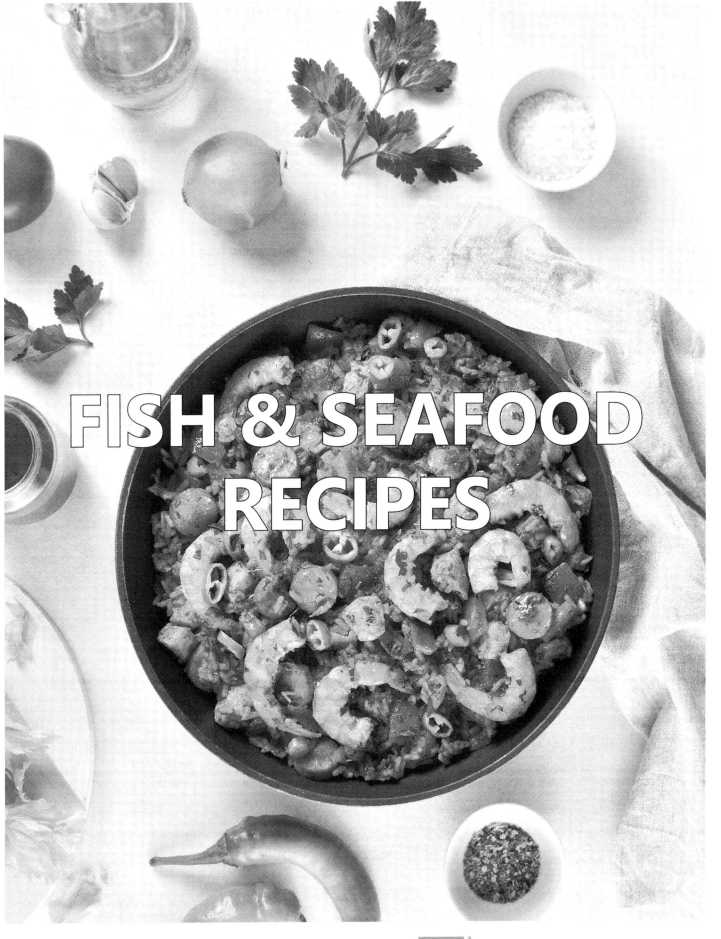

FISH & SEAFOOD RECIPES

Fish & Seafood Recipes

Sweden Fish Casserole

Servings:4
Cooking Time: 3.5 Hours

Ingredients:
- 8 oz mackerel fillet, chopped
- 1 cup of water
- 3 tablespoons mayonnaise
- 1 tablespoon sesame oil
- 1 teaspoon ground black pepper
- 2 onions, sliced
- 2 oz Provolone cheese, grated

Directions:
1. Brush the Crock Pot bottom with sesame oil.
2. Then mix chopped mackerel with onion and put in the Crock Pot.
3. Spread the mayonnaise over the fish.
4. Add grated Provolone cheese, ground black pepper, and water.
5. Close the lid and cook the casserole on High for 3.5 hours.

Nutrition Info:
- Per Serving: 295 calories, 17.9g protein, 8.4g carbohydrates, 21g fat, 1.3g fiber, 55mg cholesterol, 254mg sodium, 335mg potassium

Braised Tilapia With Capers

Servings:4
Cooking Time: 5 Hours

Ingredients:
- 4 tilapia fillets
- ½ cup of water
- 2 tablespoons sour cream
- ½ teaspoon salt
- ¼ teaspoon chili flakes
- 1 tablespoon capers

Directions:
1. Put all ingredients in the Crock Pot and close the lid.
2. Cook the tilapia on Low for 5 hours.

Nutrition Info:
- Per Serving: 106 calories, 21.3g protein, 0.4g carbohydrates, 2.3g fat, 0.1g fiber, 58mg cholesterol, 399mg sodium, 10mg potassium

Honey Mahi Mahi

Servings:4
Cooking Time: 2 Hours

Ingredients:
- 2 tablespoons of liquid honey
- 2 tablespoons butter, softened
- ½ teaspoon white pepper
- 15 oz Mahi Mahi fillet
- 1 tablespoon olive oil
- ½ cup of water

Directions:
1. Slice the fish fillet and put it in the hot skillet.
2. Add olive oil and roast the fish for 2-3 minutes per side on high heat.
3. After this, transfer the fish in the Crock Pot.
4. Add all remaining ingredients and close the lid.
5. Cook the fish on high for 2 hours.

Nutrition Info:
- Per Serving: 208 calories, 20.2g protein, 8.8g carbohydrates, 10.3g fat, 0.1g fiber, 107mg cholesterol, 178mg sodium, 404mg potassium

Cod Sticks

Servings:2
Cooking Time: 1.5 Hour

Ingredients:
- 2 cod fillets
- 1 teaspoon ground black pepper
- 1 egg, beaten
- 1/3 cup breadcrumbs
- 1 tablespoon coconut oil
- ¼ cup of water

Directions:
1. Cut the cod fillets into medium sticks and sprinkle

with ground black pepper.
2. Then dip the fish in the beaten egg and coat in the breadcrumbs.
3. Pour water in the Crock Pot.
4. Add coconut oil and fish sticks.
5. Cook the meal on High for 1.5 hours.

Nutrition Info:
• Per Serving: 254 calories, 25.3g protein, 13.8g carbohydrates, 11g fat, 1.1g fiber, 137mg cholesterol, 234mg sodium, 78mg potassium.

Cod Sticks In Blankets

Servings:4
Cooking Time: 4 Hours

Ingredients:
• 4 cod fillets
• 4 oz puff pastry
• 1 teaspoon mayonnaise
• 1 teaspoon ground black pepper
• 1 teaspoon olive oil

Directions:
1. Cut the cod fillets into the sticks.
2. Then sprinkle them with mayonnaise and ground black pepper.
3. Roll up the puff pastry and cut into strips.
4. Roll every cod stick in the puff pastry and brush with olive oil.
5. Put the cod sticks in the Crock Pot in one layer and cook on high for 4 hours.

Nutrition Info:
• Per Serving: 262 calories, 22.1g protein, 13.4g carbohydrates, 13.g fat, 0.6g fiber, 55mg cholesterol, 150mg sodium, 24mg potassium

Seafood Bean Chili

Servings: 8
Cooking Time: 3.5 Hrs.

Ingredients:
• 1 lb. salmon, diced
• 7 oz shrimps, peeled
• 1 tbsp salt
• 1 cup tomatoes, canned
• 1 tsp ground white pepper
• 1 tbsp tomato sauce
• 2 onions, chopped
• 1 cup carrot, chopped
• 1 can red beans
• ½ cup tomato juice
• 1 cup fish stock
• 1 tsp cayenne pepper
• 1 cup bell pepper, chopped
• 1 tbsp olive oil
• 1 tsp coriander
• 1 cup of water
• 6 oz Parmesan, shredded
• 1 garlic clove, sliced

Directions:
1. Add tomatoes, white pepper, tomato sauce, red beans, carrots, tomato juice, bell pepper, fish stock, cayenne pepper, garlic, water and coriander to the insert of Crock Pot.
2. Put the cooker's lid on and set the cooking time to 3 hours on High settings.
3. Add olive oil and seafood to a suitable pan, then sauté for 3 minutes.
4. Transfer the sautéed seafood to the Crock Pot.
5. Put the cooker's lid on and set the cooking time to 30 minutes on High settings.
6. Serve warm.

Nutrition Info:
• Per Serving: Calories: 281, Total Fat: 7.9g, Fiber: 4g, Total Carbs: 22.52g, Protein: 30g

Rosemary Sole

Servings:2
Cooking Time: 2 Hours

Ingredients:
• 8 oz sole fillet
• 1 tablespoon dried rosemary
• 1 tablespoon avocado oil
• 1 tablespoon apple cider vinegar
• 5 tablespoons water

Directions:
1. Pour water in the Crock Pot.
2. Then rub the sole fillet with dried rosemary and sprinkle with avocado oil and apple cider vinegar.
3. Put the fish fillet in the Crock Pot and cook it on High for 2 hours.

Nutrition Info:
• Per Serving: 149 calories, 27.6g protein, 1.5g carbohydrates, 2.9g fat, 1g fiber, 77mg cholesterol, 122mg sodium, 434mg potassium.

Cream Cheese Fish Balls

Servings:4
Cooking Time: 2 Hours

Ingredients:
- 8 oz salmon fillet, minced
- 1 tablespoon cream cheese
- ½ teaspoon dried cilantro
- ¼ teaspoon garlic powder
- 2 tablespoons flour
- ¼ cup fish stock

Directions:
1. In the mixing bowl mix minced salmon fillet with cream cheese, dried cilantro, garlic powder, and flour.
2. Make the fish balls and put them in the Crock Pot.
3. Add fish stock and close the lid.
4. Cook the meal on High for 2 hours.

Nutrition Info:
- Per Serving: 101 calories, 12g protein, 3.2g carbohydrates, 4.5g fat, 0.1g fiber, 28mg cholesterol, 55mg sodium, 248mg potassium

Crockpot Asian Shrimps

Servings:2
Cooking Time: 3 Hours

Ingredients:
- ½ cup chicken stock
- 2 tablespoons soy sauce
- ½ teaspoon sliced ginger
- ½ pound shrimps, cleaned and deveined
- 2 tablespoons rice vinegar
- 2 tablespoons sesame oil
- 2 tablespoons toasted sesame seeds
- 2 tablespoons green onions, chopped

Directions:
1. Place the chicken stock, soy sauce, ginger, shrimps, and rice vinegar in the CrockPot.
2. Give a good stir.
3. Close the lid and cook on high for 2 hours or on low for 3 hours.
4. Sprinkle with sesame oil, sesame seeds, and chopped green onions before serving.

Nutrition Info:
- Calories per serving: 352; Carbohydrates: 4.7g; Protein: 30.2g; Fat: 24.3g; Sugar: 0.4g; Sodium: 755mg; Fiber: 2.9g

Mussels And Sausage Satay

Servings: 4
Cooking Time: 2 Hrs.

Ingredients:
- 2 lbs. mussels, scrubbed and debearded
- 12 oz. amber beer
- 1 tbsp olive oil
- 1 yellow onion, chopped
- 8 oz. spicy sausage
- 1 tbsp paprika

Directions:
1. Grease the insert of your Crock Pot with oil.
2. Toss in mussels, beer, onion, sausage, and paprika.
3. Put the cooker's lid on and set the cooking time to 2 hours on High settings.
4. Discard all the unopened mussels, if any.
5. Serve the rest and enjoy it.

Nutrition Info:
- Per Serving: Calories: 124, Total Fat: 3g, Fiber: 1g, Total Carbs: 7g, Protein: 12g

Tarragon Mahi Mahi

Servings:4
Cooking Time: 2.5 Hours

Ingredients:
- 1-pound mahi-mahi fillet
- 1 tablespoon dried tarragon
- 1 tablespoon coconut oil
- ½ cup of water

Directions:
1. Melt the coconut oil in the skillet.
2. Add mahi-mahi fillet and roast it on high heat for 2 minutes per side.
3. Put the fish fillet in the Crock Pot.
4. Add dried tarragon and water.
5. Close the lid and cook the fish on High for 2.5 hours.

Nutrition Info:
- Per Serving: 121 calories, 21.2g protein, 0.2g carbohydrates, 3.4g fat, 0g fiber, 40mg cholesterol, 97mg sodium, 14mg potassium

Cod With Asparagus

Servings: 4
Cooking Time: 2 Hrs

Ingredients:
• 4 cod fillets, boneless
• 1 bunch asparagus
• 12 tbsp lemon juice
• Salt and black pepper to the taste
• 2 tbsp olive oil

Directions:
1. Place the cod fillets in separate foil sheets.
2. Top the fish with asparagus spears, lemon pepper, oil, and lemon juice.
3. Wrap the fish with its foil sheet then place them in Crock Pot.
4. Put the cooker's lid on and set the cooking time to 2 hours on High settings.
5. Unwrap the fish and serve warm.

Nutrition Info:
• Per Serving: Calories 202, Total Fat 3g, Fiber 6g, Total Carbs 7g, Protein 3g

Sea Bass And Squash

Servings: 2
Cooking Time: 3 Hours

Ingredients:
• 1 pound sea bass, boneless and cubed
• 1 cup butternut squash, peeled and cubed
• 1 teaspoon olive oil
• ½ teaspoon turmeric powder
• ½ teaspoon Italian seasoning
• 1 cup chicken stock
• 1 tablespoon cilantro, chopped

Directions:
1. In your Crock Pot, mix the sea bass with the squash, oil, turmeric and the other ingredients, toss, the lid on and cook on Low for 3 hours.
2. Divide everything between plates and serve.

Nutrition Info:
• calories 200, fat 12, fiber 3, carbs 7, protein 9

Semolina Fish Balls

Servings: 11
Cooking Time: 8 Hrs.

Ingredients:
• 1 cup sweet corn
• 5 tbsp fresh dill, chopped
• 1 tbsp minced garlic
• 7 tbsp bread crumbs
• 2 eggs, beaten
• 10 oz salmon, salmon
• 2 tbsp semolina
• 2 tbsp canola oil
• 1 tsp salt
• 1 tsp ground black pepper
• 1 tsp cumin
• 1 tsp lemon zest
• ¼ tsp cinnamon
• 3 tbsp almond flour
• 3 tbsp scallion, chopped
• 3 tbsp water

Directions:
1. Mix sweet corn, dill, garlic, semolina, eggs, salt, cumin, almond flour, scallion, cinnamon, lemon zest, and black pepper in a large bowl.
2. Stir in chopped salmon and mix well.
3. Make small meatballs out of this fish mixture then roll them in the breadcrumbs.
4. Place the coated fish ball in the insert of the Crock Pot.
5. Add canola oil and water to the fish balls.
6. Put the cooker's lid on and set the cooking time to 8 hours on Low settings.
7. Serve warm.

Nutrition Info:
• Per Serving: Calories: 201, Total Fat: 7.9g, Fiber: 2g, Total Carbs: 22.6g, Protein: 11g

Almond-crusted Tilapia

Servings:4
Cooking Time: 4 Hours

Ingredients:
• 2 tablespoons olive oil
• 1 cup chopped almonds
• ¼ cup ground flaxseed
• 4 tilapia fillets
• Salt and pepper to taste

Directions:
1. Line the bottom of the crockpot with a foil.
2. Grease the foil with the olive oil.
3. In a mixing bowl, combine the almonds and flax-seed.
4. Season the tilapia with salt and pepper to taste.
5. Dredge the tilapia fillets with the almond and flax-seed mixture.
6. Place neatly in the foil-lined crockpot.
7. Close the lid and cook on high for 2 hours and on low for 4 hours.

Nutrition Info:
- Calories per serving: 233; Carbohydrates: 4.6g; Protein: 25.5g; Fat: 13.3g; Sugar: 0.4g; Sodium: 342mg; Fiber: 1.9g

Salmon And Strawberries Mix

Servings: 2
Cooking Time: 2 Hours

Ingredients:
- 1 pound salmon fillets, boneless
- 1 cup strawberries, halved
- ½ cup orange juice
- Zest of 1 lemon, grated
- 4 scallions, chopped
- 1 teaspoon balsamic vinegar
- 1 tablespoon chives, chopped
- A pinch of salt and black pepper

Directions:
1. In your Crock Pot, mix the salmon with the strawberries, orange juice and the other ingredients, toss, put the lid on and cook on High for 2 hours.
2. Divide everything into bowls and serve.

Nutrition Info:
- calories 200, fat 12, fiber 4, carbs 6, protein 8

Mustard Salmon

Servings: 1
Cooking Time: 2 Hours

Ingredients:
- 1 big salmon fillet
- Salt and black pepper to the taste
- 2 tablespoons mustard
- 1 tablespoon olive oil
- 1 tablespoon maple extract

Directions:

1. In a bowl, mix maple extract with mustard and whisk well.
2. Season salmon with salt and pepper, brush with the mustard mix, put in your Crock Pot, cover and cook on High for 2 hours.
3. Serve the salmon with a side salad.

Nutrition Info:
- calories 240, fat 7, fiber 1, carbs 15, protein 23

Chipotle Salmon Fillets

Servings: 2
Cooking Time: 2 Hrs

Ingredients:
- 2 medium salmon fillets, boneless
- A pinch of nutmeg, ground
- A pinch of cloves, ground
- A pinch of ginger powder
- Salt and black pepper to the taste
- 2 tsp sugar
- 1 tsp onion powder
- ¼ tsp chipotle chili powder
- ½ tsp cayenne pepper
- ½ tsp cinnamon, ground
- 1/8 tsp thyme, dried

Directions:
1. Place the salmon fillets in foil wraps.
2. Drizzle ginger, cloves, salt, thyme, cinnamon, black pepper, cayenne, chili powder, onion powder, nutmeg, and coconut sugar on top.
3. Wrap the fish fillet with the aluminum foil.
4. Put the cooker's lid on and set the cooking time to 2 hours on Low settings.
5. Unwrap the fish and serve warm.

Nutrition Info:
- Per Serving: Calories 220, Total Fat 4g, Fiber 2g, Total Carbs 7g, Protein 4g

Parsley Cod

Servings: 2
Cooking Time: 2 Hours

Ingredients:
- 1 pound cod fillets, boneless
- 3 scallions, chopped
- 2 teaspoons olive oil
- Juice of 1 lime
- 1 teaspoon coriander, ground

- Salt and black pepper to the taste
- 1 tablespoon parsley, chopped

Directions:

1. In your Crock Pot, mix the cod with the scallions, the oil and the other ingredients, rub gently, put the lid on and cook on High for 1 hour.
2. Divide everything between plates and serve.

Nutrition Info:

- calories 200, fat 12, fiber 2, carbs 6, protein 9

Indian Fish

Servings: 6
Cooking Time: 2 Hours

Ingredients:

- 6 white fish fillets, cut into medium pieces
- 1 tomato, chopped
- 14 ounces coconut milk
- 2 yellow onions, sliced
- 2 red bell peppers, cut into strips
- 2 garlic cloves, minced
- 6 curry leaves
- 1 tablespoons coriander, ground
- 1 tablespoon ginger, finely grated
- ½ teaspoon turmeric, ground
- 2 teaspoons cumin, ground
- Salt and black pepper to the taste
- ½ teaspoon fenugreek, ground
- 1 teaspoon hot pepper flakes
- 2 tablespoons lemon juice

Directions:

1. In your Crock Pot, mix fish with tomato, milk, onions, bell peppers, garlic cloves, curry leaves, coriander, turmeric, cumin, salt, pepper, fenugreek, pepper flakes and lemon juice, cover and cook on High for 2 hours.
2. Toss fish, divide the whole mix between plates and serve.

Nutrition Info:

- calories 231, fat 4, fiber 6, carbs 16, protein 22

Alaska Salmon With Pecan Crunch Coating

Servings: 6
Cooking Time: 6 Hours 30 Minutes

Ingredients:

- ½ cup fresh bread crumbs

- ½ cup pecans, finely chopped
- 6 lemon wedges
- Salt and black pepper, to taste
- 3 tablespoons butter, melted
- 3 tablespoons Dijon mustard
- 5 teaspoons honey
- 6 (4 ounce) salmon fillets
- 3 teaspoons fresh parsley, chopped

Directions:

1. Season the salmon fillets with salt and black pepper and transfer into the crock pot.
2. Combine honey, mustard and butter in a small bowl.
3. Mix together the parsley, pecans and bread crumbs in another bowl.
4. Brush the salmon fillets with honey mixture and top with parsley mixture.
5. Cover and cook for about 6 hours on LOW.
6. Garnish with lemon wedges and dish out to serve warm.

Nutrition Info:

- Calories: 270 Fat: 14.4g Carbohydrates: 12.6g

Shrimps In Coconut Milk

Servings:4
Cooking Time: 3 Hours

Ingredients:

- 1-pound shrimps, shelled and deveined
- 1 tablespoon minced garlic
- 1 tablespoon grated ginger
- ½ teaspoon turmeric powder
- 1 teaspoon garam masala
- ½ teaspoon cayenne pepper
- ½ can coconut milk, unsweetened
- Salt and pepper to taste

Directions:

1. Place all ingredients in the CrockPot.
2. Give a good stir.
3. Close the lid and cook on high for 2 hours or on low for 3 hours.

Nutrition Info:

- Calories per serving: 192; Carbohydrates: 2g; Protein: 16g; Fat: 12g; Sugar: 0g; Sodium: 481mg; Fiber: 1.3g

Mackerel And Lemon

Servings: 4
Cooking Time: 2 Hours

Ingredients:
- 4 mackerels
- 3 ounces breadcrumbs
- Juice and rind of 1 lemon
- 1 tablespoon chives, finely chopped
- Salt and black pepper to the taste
- 1 egg, whisked
- 1 tablespoon butter
- 1 tablespoon vegetable oil
- 3 lemon wedges

Directions:
1. In a bowl, mix breadcrumbs with lemon juice, lemon rind, salt, pepper, egg and chives, stir very well and coat mackerel with this mix.
2. Add the oil and the butter to your Crock Pot and arrange mackerel inside.
3. Cover, cook on High for 2 hours, divide fish between plates and serve with lemon wedges on the side.

Nutrition Info:
- calories 200, fat 3, fiber 1, carbs 3, protein 12

Cod Bacon Chowder

Servings: 6
Cooking Time: 3 Hrs

Ingredients:
- 1 yellow onion, chopped
- 10 oz. cod, cubed
- 3 oz. bacon, sliced
- 1 tsp sage
- 5 oz. potatoes, peeled and cubed
- 1 carrot, grated
- 5 cups of water
- 1 tbsp almond milk
- 1 tsp ground coriander
- 1 tsp salt

Directions:
1. Place grated carrots and onion in the Crock Pot.
2. Add almond milk, coriander, water, sage, fish, potatoes, and bacon.
3. Put the cooker's lid on and set the cooking time to 3 hours on High settings.
4. Garnish with chopped parsley.
5. Serve.

Nutrition Info:
- Per Serving: Calories 108, Total Fat 4.5g, Fiber 2g, Total Carbs 8.02g, Protein 10g

Crockpot Seafood Jambalaya

Servings:7
Cooking Time: 3 Hours

Ingredients:
- 1 onion, chopped
- 2 tablespoons olive oil
- 2 ribs of celery, sliced
- 1 green bell pepper, seeded and chopped
- 1 cup tomatoes, crushed
- 1 cup chicken broth
- 2 teaspoons dried oregano
- 2 teaspoons dried parsley
- 2 teaspoons organic Cajun seasoning
- 1 teaspoon cayenne pepper
- 1-pound shrimps, shelled and deveined
- ½ pound squid, cleaned
- 2 cups grated cauliflower

Directions:
1. Place all ingredients in the CrockPot.
2. Give a good stir.
3. Close the lid and cook on high for 2 hours or on low for 3 hours.

Nutrition Info:
- Calories per serving: 205; Carbohydrates: 5.9g; Protein: 26.7g; Fat: 10.5g; Sugar: 0.2g; Sodium: 830mg; Fiber: 3.2g

Hot Salmon And Carrots

Servings: 2
Cooking Time: 3 Hours

Ingredients:
- 1 pound salmon fillets, boneless
- 1 cup baby carrots, peeled
- ½ teaspoon hot paprika
- ½ teaspoon chili powder
- ¼ cup chicken stock
- 2 scallions, chopped
- 1 tablespoon smoked paprika
- A pinch of salt and black pepper
- 2 tablespoons chives, chopped

Directions:
1. In your Crock Pot, mix the salmon with the carrots,

paprika and the other ingredients, toss, put the lid on and cook on Low for 3 hours.

2. Divide the mix between plates and serve.

Nutrition Info:
- calories 193, fat 7, fiber 3, carbs 6, protein 6

Halibut With Peach Sauce

Servings: 6
Cooking Time: 1 Hr.

Ingredients:
- 16 oz halibut fillet
- 4 tbsp peach puree
- 2 peach, pitted, peeled and chopped
- 1 tsp salt
- 1 tsp turmeric
- 1 tsp white sugar
- 1 tbsp sour cream
- ½ tsp ground white pepper
- 3 oz tangerines
- 1 tbsp maple syrup
- 1 tsp oregano
- 1 tsp olive oil
- 1 tsp garlic, sliced
- ½ tsp sage

Directions:
1. Mix the chopped peaches with peach puree, turmeric, salt, sour cream, and white sugar in a small bowl.
2. Season the halibut fillet with maple syrup, oregano, and white pepper.
3. Grease a suitable pan with olive oil and place it over medium heat.
4. Stir in sage, and sliced garlic, then sauté for 1 minute.
5. Add sage halibut to the pan and cook for 1 minute per side.
6. Pour the peach puree into the insert of the Crock Pot.
7. Add the sear halibut mixture to the peach puree.
8. Put the cooker's lid on and set the cooking time to 1 hour on Low settings.
9. Serve warm.

Nutrition Info:
- Per Serving: Calories: 198, Total Fat: 11.7g, Fiber: 1g, Total Carbs: 11.82g, Protein: 12g

Thai Style Flounder

Servings:6
Cooking Time: 6 Hours

Ingredients:
- 24 oz flounder, peeled, cleaned
- 1 lemon, sliced
- 1 teaspoon ground ginger
- ½ teaspoon cayenne pepper
- ½ teaspoon chili powder
- 1 teaspoon salt
- 1 teaspoon ground turmeric
- 1 tablespoon sesame oil
- 1 cup of water

Directions:
1. Chop the flounder roughly and put in the Crock Pot.
2. Add water and all remaining ingredients.
3. Close the lid and cook the fish on low for 6 hours.

Nutrition Info:
- Per Serving: 159 calories, 27.6g protein, 1.6g carbohydrates, 4.2g fat, 0.5g fiber, 77mg cholesterol, 511mg sodium, 425mg potassium.

LUNCH & DINNER RECIPES

Lunch & Dinner Recipes

Spring Mashed Potatoes

Servings: 4
Cooking Time: 2 1/2 Hours

Ingredients:
- 1 1/2 pounds potatoes, peeled and cubed
- 1 cup water
- Salt and pepper to taste
- 1/4 cup coconut milk
- 1 green onion, chopped
- 1 garlic clove, minced

Directions:
1. Combine the potatoes and water in your Crock Pot. Add salt and pepper and cook on high settings for 2 hours.
2. When done, puree the potatoes with a masher and stir in the coconut milk, onion and garlic.
3. Serve the mashed potatoes warm.

Herbed Risotto

Servings: 6
Cooking Time: 4 1/4 Hours

Ingredients:
- 2 tablespoons olive oil
- 1 shallot, chopped
- 1 cup white rice
- 2 cups spinach, shredded
- 2 tablespoons chopped cilantro
- 2 tablespoons chopped parsley
- 4 basil leaves, chopped
- 2 cups vegetable stock
- Salt and pepper to taste
- 1/2 cup grated Parmesan

Directions:
1. Combine the olive oil, shallot, rice, spinach, cilantro, parsley, basil, stock, salt and pepper in your Crock Pot.
2. Cook on low settings for 4 hours.
3. When done, add the Parmesan and serve the risotto warm and fresh.

Garlicky Butter Roasted Chicken

Servings: 8
Cooking Time: 8 1/4 Hours

Ingredients:
- 1 whole chicken
- 1/4 cup butter, softened
- 6 garlic cloves, minced
- 2 tablespoons chopped parsley
- 1 teaspoon dried sage
- Salt and pepper to taste
- 1/2 cup chicken stock

Directions:
1. Mix the butter, garlic, parsley, sage, salt and pepper in your crock pot.
2. Place the chicken on your working board and carefully lift up the skin on its breast and thighs, stuffing that space with the butter mixture.
3. Place the chicken in your crock pot.
4. Add the stock and cook on low settings for 8 hours.
5. Serve the chicken fresh with your favorite side dish.

Honey Apple Pork Chops

Servings: 4
Cooking Time: 5 1/4 Hours

Ingredients:
- 4 pork chops
- 2 red, tart apples, peeled, cored and cubed
- 1 shallot, chopped
- 2 garlic cloves, chopped
- 1 tablespoon olive oil
- 1 red chili, chopped
- 1 heirloom tomato, peeled and diced
- 1 cup apple cider
- 2 tablespoons honey
- Salt and pepper to taste

Directions:
1. Mix all the ingredients in your crock pot.
2. Add salt and pepper to taste and cook on low settings for 5 hours.
3. Serve the chops warm and fresh.

Vegetarian Hungarian Goulash

Servings: 8
Cooking Time: 8 1/2 Hours

Ingredients:
- 2 tablespoons olive oil
- 2 large onions, finely chopped
- 4 garlic cloves, chopped
- 2 carrots, diced
- 1 celery stalk, diced
- 1 can (15 oz.) white beans, drained
- 4 roasted red bell peppers, chopped
- 1 can fire roasted tomatoes
- 1 teaspoon smoked paprika
- 2 tablespoons tomato paste
- 2 pounds potatoes, peeled and cubed
- 2 bay leaves
- 2 cups vegetable stock
- Salt and pepper to taste

Directions:
1. Heat the oil in a skillet and add the onions. Cook for 5 minutes until softened then transfer in your crock pot,
2. Add the remaining ingredients and adjust the taste with salt and pepper.
3. Cook on low settings for 8 hours.
4. Serve the stew warm and fresh.

Spicy Beef Ragu

Servings: 6
Cooking Time: 6 1/4 Hours

Ingredients:
- 1 tablespoon canola oil
- 1 1/2 pounds ground beef
- 1 shallot, chopped
- 4 garlic cloves, chopped
- 1 teaspoon smoked paprika
- 2 tablespoons tomato paste
- 2 red bell peppers, finely chopped
- 1 cup finely chopped mushrooms
- 1 cup green peas
- 1 can fire roasted tomatoes
- 1 bay leaf
- 1 tablespoon red wine vinegar
- Salt and pepper to taste
- Grated Parmesan for serving
- Cooked spaghetti or your favorite pasta for serving

Directions:

1. Heat the oil in a skillet and add the beef. Cook for a few minutes then transfer in your crock pot.
2. Add the rest of the ingredients in the Crock Pot as well then cover and cook for 6 hours on low settings.
3. When done, serve the ragu warm with cooked pasta of your choice, preferably topped with grated Parmesan.

White Beans Stew

Servings: 10
Cooking Time: 4 Hours

Ingredients:
- 2 pounds white beans
- 3 celery stalks, chopped
- 2 carrots, chopped
- 1 bay leaf
- 1 yellow onion, chopped
- 3 garlic cloves, minced
- 1 teaspoon rosemary, dried
- 1 teaspoon oregano, dried
- 1 teaspoon thyme, dried
- 10 cups water
- Salt and black pepper to the taste
- 28 ounces canned tomatoes, chopped
- 6 cups chard, chopped

Directions:
1. In your Crock Pot, mix white beans with celery, carrots, bay leaf, onion, garlic, rosemary, oregano, thyme, water, salt, pepper, tomatoes and chard, cover and cook on High for 4 hours.
2. Stir, divide into bowls and serve for lunch,

Nutrition Info:
- calories 341, fat 8, fiber 12, carbs 20, protein 6

Tomato Sauce Beans Over Milky Grits

Servings: 6
Cooking Time: 2 1/2 Hours

Ingredients:
- 2 cans (15 oz. each) white beans, drained
- 1/4 cup sun-dried tomatoes, chopped
- 1 can fire roasted tomatoes
- 1 thyme sprig
- 1 bay leaf
- Salt and pepper to taste
- 1 1/2 cups whole milk
- 2/3 cup corn grits
- 1 tablespoon butter
- 1/2 cup grated Cheddar

Directions:
1. Combine the beans, tomatoes, thyme, bay leaf, salt and pepper in your Crock Pot.
2. Cook on high settings for 2 hours.
3. In the meantime, bring the milk to a boil and add the grits. Cook in a saucepan over low heat until the liquid is absorbed.
4. Serve the beans over cooked grits.

Fall Crock Pot Roast

Servings: 6
Cooking Time: 6 Hours

Ingredients:
- 2 sweet potatoes, cubed
- 2 carrots, chopped
- 2 pounds beef chuck roast, cubed
- ¼ cup celery, chopped
- 1 tablespoon canola oil
- 2 garlic cloves, minced
- 1 yellow onion, chopped
- 1 tablespoon flour
- 1 tablespoon brown sugar
- 1 tablespoon sugar
- 1 teaspoon cumin, ground
- Salt and black pepper to the taste
- ¾ teaspoon coriander, ground
- ½ teaspoon oregano, dried
- 1 teaspoon chili powder
- 1/8 teaspoon cinnamon powder
- ¾ teaspoon orange peel grated
- 15 ounces tomato sauce

Directions:
1. In your Crock Pot, mix potatoes with carrots, beef cubes, celery, oil, garlic, onion, flour, brown sugar, sugar, cumin, salt pepper, coriander, oregano, chili powder, cinnamon, orange peel and tomato sauce, stir, cover and cook on Low for 6 hours.
2. Divide into bowls and serve for lunch.

Nutrition Info:
- calories 278, fat 12, fiber 2, carbs 16, protein 25

Spiced Butter Chicken

Servings: 6
Cooking Time: 6 3/4 Hours

Ingredients:
- 6 chicken thighs
- 2 tablespoons butter
- 1 large onion, chopped
- 4 garlic cloves, chopped
- 1 teaspoon curry powder
- 1 teaspoon garam masala
- 1/2 teaspoon cumin powder
- 1/4 teaspoon chili powder
- 1 1/2 cups coconut milk
- Salt and pepper to taste
- 1/2 cup plain yogurt for serving

Directions:
1. Heat the butter in your Crock Pot. Add the chicken and cook on all sides until golden brown.
2. Transfer the chicken in your Crock Pot and add the remaining ingredients.
3. Cook on low settings for 6 hours.
4. Serve the chicken warm and fresh.

Cashew Chicken

Servings: 6
Cooking Time: 4 1/4 Hours

Ingredients:
- 3 chicken breasts, cut into strips
- 1 shallot, sliced
- 1 celery stalk, sliced
- 1 head broccoli, cut into florets
- 1 cup cashew nuts, soaked overnight
- 1/2 teaspoon ginger powder
- 1 cup chicken stock
- Salt and pepper to taste

Directions:
1. Combine the chicken, shallot, celery and broccoli in your crock pot.
2. Mix the cashew nuts, ginger and stock in a blender. Pulse until smooth then pour this mixture over the chicken in the pot.
3. Season with salt and pepper.
4. Cook on low settings for 4 hours.
5. Serve the chicken warm and fresh.

Cowboy Beef

Servings: 6
Cooking Time: 6 1/4 Hours

Ingredients:
- 2 1/2 pounds beef sirloin roast
- 6 bacon slices, chopped
- 2 onions, sliced
- 4 garlic cloves, chopped
- 1 can (15 oz.) red beans, drained
- 1 cup BBQ sauce
- 1 teaspoon chili powder
- Salt and pepper to taste
- Coleslaw for serving

Directions:
1. Mix the beef sirloin, bacon, onions, garlic, red beans, BBQ sauce, chili powder, salt and pepper and cover with a lid.
2. Cook on low settings for 6 hours.
3. Serve the beef warm and fresh, topped with fresh coleslaw.

Teriyaki Pork

Servings: 8
Cooking Time: 7 Hours

Ingredients:
- 2 tablespoons sugar
- 2 tablespoons soy sauce
- ¾ cup apple juice
- 1 teaspoon ginger powder
- 1 tablespoon white vinegar
- Salt and black pepper to the taste
- ¼ teaspoon garlic powder
- 3 pounds pork loin roast, halved
- 7 teaspoons cornstarch
- 3 tablespoons water

Directions:
1. In your Crock Pot, mix apple juice with sugar, soy sauce, vinegar, ginger, garlic powder, salt, pepper and pork loin, toss well, cover and cook on Low for 7 hours.
2. Transfer cooking juices to a small pan, heat up over medium-high heat, add cornstarch mixed with water, stir well, cook for 2 minutes until it thickens and take off heat.
3. Slice roast, divide between plates, drizzle sauce all over and serve for lunch.

Nutrition Info:
- calories 247, fat 8, fiber 1, carbs 9, protein 33

Parsley Chicken Stew

Servings: 2
Cooking Time: 4 Hours

Ingredients:
- 1 tablespoon olive oil
- Salt and black pepper to the taste
- 2 spring onions, chopped
- 1 carrot, peeled and sliced
- ¼ cup chicken stock
- 1 pound chicken breast, skinless, boneless sand cubed
- ½ cup tomato sauce
- 1 tablespoon parsley, chopped

Directions:
1. In your Crock Pot, mix the chicken with the spring onions and the other ingredients, toss, put the lid on and cook on High for 4 hours.
2. Divide into bowls and serve.

Nutrition Info:
- calories 453, fat 15, fiber 5, carbs 20, protein 20

Button Mushroom Beef Stew

Servings: 6
Cooking Time: 6 1/2 Hours

Ingredients:
- 2 pounds beef roast, cubed
- 1 tablespoon all-purpose flour
- 2 tablespoons canola oil
- 2 carrots, diced
- 1 celery root, peeled and diced
- 1 can fire roasted tomatoes
- 1 pound button mushrooms
- 1 cup beef stock
- 2 bay leaves
- 1 red chili, chopped
- Salt and pepper to taste

Directions:
1. Season the beef with salt and pepper and sprinkle it with flour.
2. Heat the oil in a frying pan and add the beef. Cook for a few minutes until golden then transfer in your Crock Pot.
3. Add the rest of the ingredients and adjust the taste with salt and pepper.
4. Cover and cook on low settings for 6 hours.
5. Serve the stew warm or chilled.

Orange Marmalade Glazed Carrots

Servings: 4
Cooking Time: 4 1/4 Hours

Ingredients:
- 20 oz. baby carrots
- 1/4 cup orange marmalade
- 1/4 teaspoon chili powder
- 1 pinch nutmeg
- 2 tablespoons water
- 1/4 teaspoon cumin powder
- Salt and pepper to taste

Directions:
1. Combine the carrots and the remaining ingredients in your Crock Pot.
2. Add salt and pepper and cover with a lid.
3. Cook on low settings for 4 hours.
4. Serve the glazed carrots warm or chilled.

Beans And Pumpkin Chili

Servings: 10
Cooking Time: 4 Hours

Ingredients:
- 1 yellow bell pepper, chopped
- 1 yellow onion, chopped
- 3 garlic cloves, minced
- 2 tablespoons olive oil
- 3 cups chicken stock
- 30 ounces canned black beans, drained
- 14 ounces pumpkin, cubed
- 2 and ½ cups turkey meat, cooked and cubed
- 2 teaspoons parsley, dried
- 1 and ½ teaspoon oregano, dried
- 2 teaspoons chili powder
- 1 and ½ teaspoon cumin, ground
- Salt and black pepper to the taste

Directions:
1. Heat up a pan with the oil over medium-high heat, add bell pepper, onion and garlic, stir, cook for a few minutes and transfer to your Crock Pot.
2. Add stock, beans, pumpkin, turkey, parsley, oregano, chili powder, cumin, salt and pepper, stir, cover and cook on Low for 4 hours.
3. Divide into bowls and serve right away for lunch.

Nutrition Info:
- calories 200, fat 5, fiber 7, carbs 20, protein 15

Chicken Cauliflower Gratin

Servings: 6
Cooking Time: 6 1/4 Hours

Ingredients:
- 1 head cauliflower, cut into florets
- 2 chicken breasts, cubed
- 1/2 teaspoon garlic powder
- 1 pinch cayenne pepper
- 1 can condensed cream of chicken soup
- Salt and pepper to taste
- 1 1/2 cups grated Cheddar

Directions:
1. Combine the cauliflower, chicken, garlic powder, cayenne pepper, chicken soup, salt and pepper in your crock pot.
2. Top with grated cheese and cook on low settings for 6 hours.
3. Serve the gratin warm and fresh.

Roasted Bell Pepper Pork Stew

Servings: 6
Cooking Time: 5 1/4 Hours

Ingredients:
- 2 pounds pork tenderloin, cubed
- 2 tablespoons canola oil
- 1 jar roasted bell pepper, drained and chopped
- 4 garlic cloves, chopped
- 1 large onion, chopped
- 1/2 teaspoon red pepper flakes
- 1 cup chicken stock
- 1 cup tomato sauce
- Salt and pepper to taste

Directions:
1. Heat the oil in a skillet and add the pork. Cook for a few minutes on all sides until golden. Transfer in your Crock Pot.
2. Add the rest of the ingredients and adjust the taste with salt and pepper.
3. Cover the pot with its lid and cook on low settings for 5 hours.
4. Serve the stew warm or chilled.

Layered Spinach Ricotta Lasagna

Servings: 10
Cooking Time: 6 1/2 Hours

Ingredients:
- 16 oz. frozen spinach, thawed
- 1 cup ricotta cheese
- 1/2 teaspoon dried marjoram
- 1/2 teaspoon dried basil
- 2 garlic cloves, chopped
- 1/2 cup grated Parmesan
- 2 1/2 cups tomato sauce
- Salt and pepper to taste
- 6 lasagna noodles
- 2 cups shredded mozzarella cheese

Directions:
1. Mix the spinach, ricotta, marjoram, basil, garlic, parmesan, salt and pepper in a bowl.
2. Begin layering the lasagna noodles, spinach and ricotta filling and the tomato sauce in your Crock Pot.
3. Top with shredded mozzarella and cook on low settings for 6 hours.
4. Serve the lasagna warm.

Hoisin Tofu

Servings: 6
Cooking Time: 6 1/4 Hours

Ingredients:
- 12 oz. firm tofu, sliced
- 1/4 cup smooth peanut butter
- 1/4 cup soy sauce
- 2 tablespoons canola oil
- 2 garlic cloves
- 1/4 teaspoon chili powder
- 1/4 teaspoon cumin powder
- 1/2 cup water

Directions:
1. Combine the peanut butter, soy sauce, canola oil, garlic, chili powder, cumin powder and water in your blender. Pulse until smooth.
2. Mix the tofu and sauce in your crock pot.
3. Cover and cook on low settings for 6 hours.
4. Serve the tofu warm with your favorite side dish.

Hominy Beef Chili

Servings: 6
Cooking Time: 3 1/4 Hours

Ingredients:
- 1 pound ground beef
- 1 large onion, chopped
- 4 garlic cloves, chopped
- 2 carrots, diced
- 2 red bell peppers, cored and diced
- 1 can (15 oz.) hominy, drained
- 1 can fire roasted tomatoes
- 2 jalapeno peppers, chopped
- 1/2 teaspoon cumin powder
- 1 teaspoon chili powder
- 2 cups frozen corn
- Salt and pepper to taste
- 1 bay leaf
- Grated Cheddar for serving

Directions:
1. Mix the ground beef, onion, garlic, carrots, bell peppers, hominy, tomatoes, jalapeno peppers, cumin powder, chili powder and corn in your crock pot.
2. Add the bay leaf, salt and pepper to taste and cook on high settings for 3 hours.
3. Serve the chili warm, topped with grated Cheddar.

Orange Beef Dish

Servings: 5
Cooking Time: 5 Hours

Ingredients:
- 1 pound beef sirloin steak, cut into medium strips
- 2 and ½ cups shiitake mushrooms, sliced
- 1 yellow onion, cut into medium wedges
- 3 red hot chilies, dried
- ¼ cup brown sugar
- ¼ cup orange juice
- ¼ cup soy sauce
- 2 tablespoons cider vinegar
- 1 tablespoon cornstarch
- 1 tablespoon ginger, grated
- 1 tablespoon sesame oil
- 1 cup snow peas
- 2 garlic cloves, minced
- 1 tablespoon orange zest, grated

Directions:
1. In your Crock Pot, mix steak strips with mushrooms, onion, chilies, sugar, orange juice, soy sauce, vinegar, cornstarch, ginger, oil, garlic and orange zest, toss, cover and cook on Low for 4 hours and 30 minutes.
2. Add snow peas, cover, cook on Low for 30 minutes more, divide between plates and serve.

Nutrition Info:
- calories 310, fat 7, fiber 4, carbs 26, protein 33

Tangy Pomegranate Beef Short Ribs

Servings: 6
Cooking Time: 6 1/4 Hours

Ingredients:
- 4 pounds beef short ribs
- 2 tablespoons olive oil
- 1 large onion, sliced
- 2 carrots, sliced
- 2 tablespoons brown sugar
- 1 cup fresh pomegranate juice
- 1/2 cup pomegranate kernels
- 1/4 cup low sodium soy sauce
- 1 teaspoon Worcestershire sauce
- 1 teaspoon dried thyme
- 1 rosemary sprig

Directions:
1. Combine all the ingredients in a Crock Pot.
2. Cover the pot with its lid and cook on low settings for 6 hours.
3. Serve the short ribs warm and sticky.

Chicken Pilaf

Servings:3
Cooking Time: 6 Hours

Ingredients:
- ½ cup basmati rice
- 2 cups of water
- 5 oz chicken fillet, chopped
- 1 teaspoon chili powder
- ½ teaspoon salt

Directions:
1. Put the rice and chicken fillet in the Crock Pot.
2. Add chili powder, salt, and water. Carefully stir the ingredients and close the lid.
3. Cook the pilaf on Low for 6 hours.

Nutrition Info:
- Per Serving: 205 calories, 16g protein, 25.1g carbohydrates, 3.9g fat, 0.7g fiber, 42mg cholesterol, 443mg

sodium, 169mg potassium.

Tofu Ratatouille

Servings: 6
Cooking Time: 3 1/2 Hours

Ingredients:
- 10 oz. firm tofu, cubed
- 2 tablespoons olive oil
- 1 teaspoon cumin powder
- 1 small eggplant, peeled and cubed
- 1 red onion, chopped
- 2 ripe tomatoes, peeled and diced
- 1 carrot, diced
- 2 red bell peppers, cored and diced
- 1 zucchini, cubed
- 1/2 teaspoon dried oregano
- Salt and pepper to taste

Directions:
1. Season the tofu with cumin powder, salt and pepper if needed.
2. Heat the oil in a skillet and add the tofu. Cook on all sides until golden then transfer in your crock pot.
3. Add the rest of the ingredients and cook on high settings for 3 hours.
4. Serve the dish warm when it's done.

Tomato Crouton Stew

Servings: 6
Cooking Time: 6 1/4 Hours

Ingredients:
- 4 ripe heirloom tomatoes, peeled and cubed
- 2 sweet onions, chopped
- 2 tablespoons olive oil
- 2 garlic cloves, chopped
- 2 red bell peppers, cored and diced
- 2 tablespoons tomato paste
- 1 1/2 cups vegetable stock
- 4 cups bread croutons
- Salt and pepper to taste
- 1/2 teaspoon dried thyme
- 1/2 teaspoon dried oregano

Directions:
1. Heat the oil in a skillet and add the onions and garlic. Cook on low settings for 2 minutes until softened then transfer in your Crock Pot.
2. Add the remaining ingredients and season with salt and pepper.

3. Cook on low settings for 6 hours.
4. Serve the stew warm and fresh.

Fruity Veal Shanks

Servings: 4
Cooking Time: 3 1/4 Hours

Ingredients:
- 4 veal shanks
- 1 orange, zested and juiced
- 1/2 cup dried apricots, chopped
- 1/4 cup dried cranberries
- 1 cup beef stock
- 1 cup diced tomatoes
- 1 rosemary sprig
- 1 thyme sprig
- Salt and pepper to taste
- 2 sweet potatoes, peeled and cubed

Directions:
1. Season the veal shanks with salt and pepper.
2. Mix the orange juice, orange zest, apricots, cranberries, stock, tomatoes, rosemary and thyme in your crock pot.
3. Add salt, pepper and the sweet potatoes and cook for 3 hours on high settings.
4. The dish is best served warm, but it can also be re-heated.

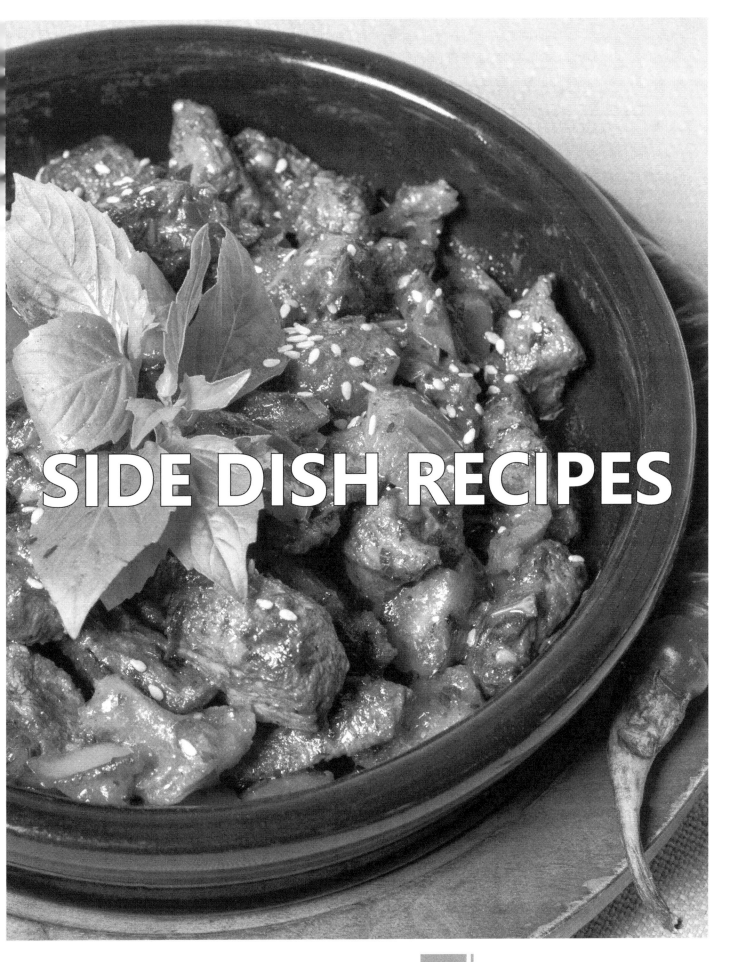

SIDE DISH RECIPES

Summer Squash Medley

Servings: 4
Cooking Time: 2 Hrs

Ingredients:
- ¼ cup olive oil
- 2 tbsp basil, chopped
- 2 tbsp balsamic vinegar
- 2 garlic cloves, minced
- 2 tsp mustard
- Salt and black pepper to the taste
- 3 summer squash, sliced
- 2 zucchinis, sliced

Directions:
1. Add squash, zucchinis, and all other ingredients to the Crock Pot.
2. Put the cooker's lid on and set the cooking time to 2 hours on High settings.
3. Serve.

Nutrition Info:
- Per Serving: Calories: 179, Total Fat: 13g, Fiber: 2g, Total Carbs: 10g, Protein: 4g

Chicken With Sweet Potato

Servings: 6
Cooking Time: 3 Hours

Ingredients:
- 16 oz. sweet potato, peeled and diced
- 3 cups chicken stock
- 1 tbsp salt
- 3 tbsp margarine
- 2 tbsp cream cheese

Directions:
1. Add sweet potato, chicken stock, and salt to the Crock Pot.
2. Put the cooker's lid on and set the cooking time to 5 hours on High settings.
3. Drain the slow-cooked potatoes and transfer them to a suitable bowl.
4. Mash the sweet potatoes and stir in cream cheese

and margarine.
5. Serve fresh.

Nutrition Info:
- Per Serving: Calories: 472, Total Fat: 31.9g, Fiber: 6.7g, Total Carbs: 43.55g, Protein: 3g

Mashed Potatoes

Servings: 2
Cooking Time: 6 Hours

Ingredients:
- 1 pound gold potatoes, peeled and cubed
- 2 garlic cloves, chopped
- 1 cup milk
- 1 cup water
- 2 tablespoons butter
- A pinch of salt and white pepper

Directions:
1. In your Crock Pot, mix the potatoes with the water, salt and pepper, put the lid on and cook on Low for 6 hours.
2. Mash the potatoes, add the rest of the ingredients, whisk and serve.

Nutrition Info:
- calories 135, fat 4, fiber 2, carbs 10, protein 4

Mashed Potatoes

Servings: 12
Cooking Time: 4 Hours

Ingredients:
- 3 pounds gold potatoes, peeled and cubed
- 1 bay leaf
- 6 garlic cloves, minced
- 28 ounces chicken stock
- 1 cup milk
- ¼ cup butter
- Salt and black pepper to the taste

Directions:
1. In your Crock Pot, mix potatoes with bay leaf, garlic, salt, pepper and stock, cover and cook on Low for

4 hours.
2. Drain potatoes, mash them, mix with butter and milk, blend really, divide between plates and serve as a side dish.

Nutrition Info:
- calories 135, fat 4, fiber 2, carbs 22, protein 4

Apples And Potatoes

Servings: 10
Cooking Time: 7 Hours

Ingredients:
- 2 green apples, cored and cut into wedges
- 3 pounds sweet potatoes, peeled and cut into medium wedges
- 1 cup coconut cream
- ½ cup dried cherries
- 1 cup apple butter
- 1 and ½ teaspoon pumpkin pie spice

Directions:
1. In your Crock Pot, mix sweet potatoes with green apples, cream, cherries, apple butter and spice, toss, cover and cook on Low for 7 hours.
2. Toss, divide between plates and serve as a side dish.

Nutrition Info:
- calories 351, fat 8, fiber 5, carbs 48, protein 2

Chorizo And Cauliflower Mix

Servings: 4
Cooking Time: 5 Hours

Ingredients:
- 1 pound chorizo, chopped
- 12 ounces canned green chilies, chopped
- 1 yellow onion, chopped
- ½ teaspoon garlic powder
- Salt and black pepper to the taste
- 1 cauliflower head, riced
- 2 tablespoons green onions, chopped

Directions:
1. Heat up a pan over medium heat, add chorizo and onion, stir, brown for a few minutes and transfer to your Crock Pot.
2. Add chilies, garlic powder, salt, pepper, cauliflower and green onions, toss, cover and cook on Low for 5 hours.
3. Divide between plates and serve as a side dish.

Nutrition Info:
- calories 350, fat 12, fiber 4, carbs 6, protein 20

Butternut Squash And Eggplant Mix

Servings: 2
Cooking Time: 4 Hours

Ingredients:
- 1 butternut squash, peeled and roughly cubed
- 1 eggplant, roughly cubed
- 1 red onion, chopped
- Cooking spray
- ½ cup veggie stock
- ¼ cup tomato paste
- ½ tablespoon parsley, chopped
- Salt and black pepper to the taste
- 2 garlic cloves, minced

Directions:
1. Grease the Crock Pot with the cooking spray and mix the squash with the eggplant, onion and the other ingredients inside.
2. Put the lid on and cook on Low for 4 hours.
3. Divide between plates and serve as a side dish.

Nutrition Info:
- calories 114, fat 4, fiber 4, carbs 18, protein 4

Coconut Bok Choy

Servings: 2
Cooking Time: 1 Hour

Ingredients:
- 1 pound bok choy, torn
- ½ cup chicken stock
- ½ teaspoon chili powder
- 1 garlic clove, minced
- 1 teaspoon ginger, grated
- 1 tablespoon coconut oil
- Salt to the taste

Directions:
1. In your Crock Pot, mix the bok choy with the stock and the other ingredients, toss, put the lid on and cook on High for 1 hour.
2. Divide between plates and serve as a side dish.

Nutrition Info:
- calories 100, fat 1, fiber 2, carbs 7, protein 4

Bacon Potatoes Mix

Servings: 2
Cooking Time: 6 Hours

Ingredients:

- 2 sweet potatoes, peeled and cut into wedges
- 1 tablespoon balsamic vinegar
- ½ tablespoon sugar
- A pinch of salt and black pepper
- ¼ teaspoon sage, dried
- A pinch of thyme, dried
- 1 tablespoon olive oil
- ½ cup veggie stock
- 2 bacon slices, cooked and crumbled

Directions:

1. In your Crock Pot, mix the potatoes with the vinegar, sugar and the other ingredients, toss, put the lid on and cook on Low for 6 hours
2. Divide between plates and serve as a side dish.

Nutrition Info:

- calories 209, fat 4, fiber 4, carbs 29, protein 4

Maple Brussels Sprouts

Servings: 12
Cooking Time: 3 Hours

Ingredients:

- 1 cup red onion, chopped
- 2 pounds Brussels sprouts, trimmed and halved
- Salt and black pepper to the taste
- ¼ cup apple juice
- 3 tablespoons olive oil
- ¼ cup maple syrup
- 1 tablespoon thyme, chopped

Directions:

1. In your Crock Pot, mix Brussels sprouts with onion, salt, pepper and apple juice, toss, cover and cook on Low for 3 hours.
2. In a bowl, mix maple syrup with oil and thyme, whisk really well, add over Brussels sprouts, toss well, divide between plates and serve as a side dish.

Nutrition Info:

- calories 100, fat 4, fiber 4, carbs 14, protein 3

Cauliflower And Broccoli Mix

Servings: 10
Cooking Time: 7 Hours

Ingredients:

- 4 cups broccoli florets
- 4 cups cauliflower florets
- 7 ounces Swiss cheese, torn
- 14 ounces Alfredo sauce
- 1 yellow onion, chopped
- Salt and black pepper to the taste
- 1 teaspoon thyme, dried
- ½ cup almonds, sliced

Directions:

1. In your Crock Pot, mix broccoli with cauliflower, cheese, sauce, onion, salt, pepper and thyme, stir, cover and cook on Low for 7 hours.
2. Add almonds, divide between plates and serve as a side dish.

Nutrition Info:

- calories 177, fat 7, fiber 2, carbs 10, protein 7

Sage Peas

Servings: 2
Cooking Time: 2 Hours

Ingredients:

- 1 pound peas
- 1 red onion, sliced
- ½ cup veggie stock
- ½ cup tomato sauce
- 2 garlic cloves, minced
- ¼ teaspoon sage, dried
- Salt and black pepper to the taste
- 1 tablespoon dill, chopped

Directions:

1. In your Crock Pot, combine the peas with the onion, stock and the other ingredients, toss, put the lid on and cook on Low for 2 hours.
2. Divide between plates and serve as a side dish.

Nutrition Info:

- calories 100, fat 4, fiber 3, carbs 15, protein 4

Herbed Beets

Servings: 4
Cooking Time: 7 Hours

Ingredients:
- 6 medium assorted-color beets, peeled and cut into wedges
- 2 tablespoons balsamic vinegar
- 2 tablespoons olive oil
- 2 tablespoons chives, chopped
- 1 tablespoon tarragon, chopped
- Salt and black pepper to the taste
- 1 teaspoon orange peel, grated

Directions:
1. In your Crock Pot, mix beets with vinegar, oil, chives, tarragon, salt, pepper and orange peel, cover and cook on Low for 7 hours.
2. Divide between plates and serve as a side dish.

Nutrition Info:
- calories 144, fat 3, fiber 1, carbs 17, protein 3

Beans And Red Peppers

Servings: 2
Cooking Time: 2 Hrs.

Ingredients:
- 2 cups green beans, halved
- 1 red bell pepper, cut into strips
- Salt and black pepper to the taste
- 1 tbsp olive oil
- 1 and ½ tbsp honey mustard

Directions:
1. Add green beans, honey mustard, red bell pepper, oil, salt, and black to Crock Pot.
2. Put the cooker's lid on and set the cooking time to 2 hours on High settings.
3. Serve warm.

Nutrition Info:
- Per Serving: Calories: 50, Total Fat: 0g, Fiber: 4g, Total Carbs: 8g, Protein: 2g

Orange Glazed Carrots

Servings: 10
Cooking Time: 8 Hours

Ingredients:
- 3 pounds carrots, cut into medium chunks
- 1 cup orange juice
- 2 tablespoons orange peel, grated
- ½ cup orange marmalade
- ½ cup veggie stock
- ¼ cup white wine
- 1 tablespoon tapioca, crushed
- ¼ cup parsley, chopped
- 3 tablespoons butter
- Salt and black pepper to the taste

Directions:
1. In your Crock Pot, mix carrots with orange juice, orange peel, marmalade, stock, wine, tapioca, parsley, butter, salt and pepper, cover and cook on Low for 8 hours.
2. Toss carrots, divide between plates and serve as a side dish.

Nutrition Info:
- calories 160, fat 4, fiber 4, carbs 31, protein 3

Jalapeno Meal

Servings: 6
Cooking Time: 6 Hrs.

Ingredients:
- 12 oz. jalapeno pepper, cut in half and deseeded
- 2 tbsp olive oil
- 1 tbsp balsamic vinegar
- 1 onion, sliced
- 1 garlic clove, sliced
- 1 tsp ground coriander
- 4 tbsp water

Directions:
1. Place the jalapeno peppers in the Crock Pot.
2. Top the pepper with olive oil, balsamic vinegar, onion, garlic, coriander, and water.
3. Put the cooker's lid on and set the cooking time to 6 hours on Low settings.
4. Serve warm.

Nutrition Info:
- Per Serving: Calories: 67, Total Fat: 4.7g, Fiber: 2g, Total Carbs: 6.02g, Protein: 1g

Hot Zucchini Mix

Servings: 2
Cooking Time: 2 Hours

Ingredients:
- ¼ cup carrots, grated
- 1 pound zucchinis, roughly cubed
- 1 teaspoon hot paprika
- ½ teaspoon chili powder
- 2 spring onions, chopped
- ½ tablespoon olive oil
- ½ teaspoon curry powder
- 1 garlic clove, minced
- ½ teaspoon ginger powder
- A pinch of salt and black pepper
- 1 tablespoon cilantro, chopped

Directions:
1. In your Crock Pot, mix the carrots with the zucchinis, paprika and the other ingredients, toss, put the lid on and cook on Low for 2 hours.
2. Divide between plates and serve as a side dish.

Nutrition Info:
- calories 200, fat 5, fiber 7, carbs 28, protein 4

Tangy Red Potatoes

Servings: 4
Cooking Time: 8 Hours

Ingredients:
- 1 lb. red potato
- 2 tbsp olive oil
- 1 garlic clove
- 1 tsp sage
- 4 tbsp mayo
- 1 tsp minced garlic
- 3 tbsp fresh dill, chopped
- 1 tsp paprika

Directions:
1. Add potatoes, olive oil, garlic cloves, garlic, and sage to the Crock Pot.
2. Put the cooker's lid on and set the cooking time to 8 hours on Low settings.
3. Whisk mayo and minced garlic in a suitable bowl.
4. Transfer the slow-cooked potatoes to a bowl and mash them using a fork.
5. Stir in the mayo-garlic mixture then mix well.
6. Serve fresh.

Nutrition Info:

- Per Serving: Calories: 164, Total Fat: 7.8g, Fiber: 4g, Total Carbs: 22.87g, Protein: 3g

Saucy Macaroni

Servings: 6
Cooking Time: 3.5 Hours

Ingredients:
- 8 oz. macaroni
- 1 cup tomatoes, chopped
- 1 garlic clove, peeled
- 1 tsp butter
- 1 cup heavy cream
- 3 cups of water
- 1 tbsp salt
- 6 oz. Parmesan, shredded
- 1 tbsp dried basil

Directions:
1. Add macaroni, salt, and water to the Crock Pot.
2. Put the cooker's lid on and set the cooking time to 3 hours on High settings.
3. Meanwhile, puree tomatoes in a blender then add cheese, cream, butter, and dried basil.
4. Drain the cooked macaroni and return them to the Crock Pot.
5. Pour in the tomato-cream mixture.
6. Put the cooker's lid on and set the cooking time to 30 minutes on High settings.
7. Serve warm.

Nutrition Info:
- Per Serving: Calories: 325, Total Fat: 10.1g, Fiber: 2g, Total Carbs: 41.27g, Protein: 17g

Slow-cooked White Onions

Servings: 5
Cooking Time: 9 Hours

Ingredients:

- ½ cup bread crumbs
- 5 oz. Romano cheese, shredded
- ¼ cup cream cheese
- ¼ cup half and half
- 3 oz. butter
- 1 tbsp salt
- 5 large white onions, peeled and wedges
- 1 tsp ground black pepper
- 1 tsp garlic powder

Directions:

1. Add onion wedges to the insert of the Crock Pot.
2. Mix breadcrumbs and shredded cheese in a suitable bowl.
3. Whisk the half and half cream with remaining ingredients.
4. Spread this mixture over the onion and then top it with breadcrumbs mixture.
5. Put the cooker's lid on and set the cooking time to 9 hours on Low settings.
6. Serve warm.

Nutrition Info:

- Per Serving: Calories: 349, Total Fat: 25.3g, Fiber: 3g, Total Carbs: 19.55g, Protein: 13g

Beans, Carrots And Spinach Salad

Servings: 6
Cooking Time: 7 Hours

Ingredients:

- 1 and ½ cups northern beans
- 1 yellow onion, chopped
- 5 carrots, chopped
- 2 garlic cloves, minced
- ½ teaspoon oregano, dried
- Salt and black pepper to the taste
- 4 and ½ cups chicken stock
- 5 ounces baby spinach
- 2 teaspoons lemon peel, grated
- 1 avocado, peeled, pitted and chopped
- 3 tablespoons lemon juice
- ¾ cup feta cheese, crumbled
- 1/3 cup pistachios, chopped

Directions:

1. In your Crock Pot, mix beans with onion, carrots, garlic, oregano, salt, pepper and stock, stir, cover and cook on Low for 7 hours.
2. Drain beans and veggies, transfer them to a salad bowl, add baby spinach, lemon peel, avocado, lemon juice, pistachios and cheese, toss, divide between plates and serve as a side dish.

Nutrition Info:

- calories 300, fat 8, fiber 14, carbs 43, protein 16

Rice And Artichokes

Servings: 4
Cooking Time: 4 Hours

Ingredients:

- 1 tablespoon olive oil
- 5 ounces Arborio rice
- 2 garlic cloves, minced
- 1 and ¼ cups chicken stock
- 1 tablespoon white wine
- 6 ounces graham crackers, crumbled
- 1 and ¼ cups water
- 15 ounces canned artichoke hearts, chopped
- 16 ounces cream cheese
- 1 tablespoon parmesan, grated
- 1 and ½ tablespoons thyme, chopped
- Salt and black pepper to the taste

Directions:

1. In your Crock Pot, mix oil with rice, garlic, stock, wine, water, artichokes and crackers, stir, cover and cook on Low for 4 hours.
2. Add cream cheese, salt, pepper, parmesan and thyme, toss, divide between plates and serve as a side dish.

Nutrition Info:

- calories 230, fat 3, fiber 5, carbs 30, protein 4

Cauliflower And Almonds Mix

Servings: 2
Cooking Time: 3 Hours

Ingredients:
- 2 cups cauliflower florets
- 2 ounces tomato paste
- 1 small yellow onion, chopped
- 1 tablespoon chives, chopped
- Salt and black pepper to the taste
- 1 tablespoon almonds, sliced

Directions:
1. In your Crock Pot, mix the cauliflower with the tomato paste and the other ingredients, toss, put the lid on and cook on High for 3 hours.
2. Divide between plates and serve as a side dish.

Nutrition Info:
- calories 177, fat 12, fiber 7, carbs 20, protein 7

Mexican Rice

Servings: 8
Cooking Time: 4 Hours

Ingredients:
- 1 cup long grain rice
- 1 and ¼ cups veggie stock
- ½ cup cilantro, chopped
- ½ avocado, pitted, peeled and chopped
- Salt and black pepper to the taste
- ¼ cup green hot sauce

Directions:
1. Put the rice in your Crock Pot, add stock, stir, cover, cook on Low for 4 hours, fluff with a fork and transfer to a bowl.
2. In your food processor, mix avocado with hot sauce and cilantro, blend well, pour over rice, toss well, add salt and pepper, divide between plates and serve as a side dish.

Nutrition Info:
- calories 100, fat 3, fiber 6, carbs 18, protein 4

Refried Black Beans

Servings: 10
Cooking Time: 9 Hours

Ingredients:
- 5 oz. white onion, peeled and chopped
- 4 cups black beans
- 1 chili pepper, chopped
- 1 oz. minced garlic
- 10 cups water
- 1 tsp salt
- ½ tsp ground black pepper
- ¼ tsp cilantro, chopped

Directions:
1. Add onion, black beans and all other ingredients to the Crock Pot.
2. Put the cooker's lid on and set the cooking time to 9 hours on Low settings.
3. Strain all the excess liquid out of the beans while leaving only ¼ cup of the liquid.
4. Transfer the beans-onion mixture to a food processor and blend until smooth.
5. Serve fresh.

Nutrition Info:
- Per Serving: Calories: 73, Total Fat: 1.5g, Fiber: 4g, Total Carbs: 12.34g, Protein: 3g

Mustard Brussels Sprouts(2)

Servings: 2
Cooking Time: 3 Hours

Ingredients:
- ½ pounds Brussels sprouts, trimmed and halved
- A pinch of salt and black pepper
- 2 tablespoons mustard
- ½ cup veggie stock
- 1 tablespoons olive oil
- 2 tablespoons maple syrup
- 1 tablespoon thyme, chopped

Directions:
1. In your Crock Pot, mix the sprouts with the mustard and the other ingredients, toss, put the lid on and cook on Low for 3 hours.
2. Divide between plates and serve as a side dish.

Nutrition Info:
- calories 170, fat 4, fiber 4, carbs 14, protein 6

Baby Carrots And Parsnips Mix

Servings: 2
Cooking Time: 6 Hours

Ingredients:
- 1 tablespoon avocado oil
- 1 pound baby carrots, peeled
- ½ pound parsnips, peeled and cut into sticks
- 1 teaspoon sweet paprika
- ½ cup tomato paste
- ½ cup veggie stock
- ½ teaspoon chili powder
- A pinch of salt and black pepper
- 2 garlic cloves, minced
- 1 tablespoon dill, chopped

Directions:
1. Grease the Crock Pot with the oil and mix the carrots with the parsnips, paprika and the other ingredients inside.
2. Toss, put the lid on and cook on Low for 6 hours.
3. Divide everything between plates and serve as a side dish.

Nutrition Info:
- calories 273, fat 7, fiber 5, carbs 8, protein 12

Okra And Corn

Servings: 4
Cooking Time: 8 Hours

Ingredients:
- 3 garlic cloves, minced
- 1 small green bell pepper, chopped
- 1 small yellow onion, chopped
- 1 cup water
- 16 ounces okra, sliced
- 2 cups corn
- 1 and ½ teaspoon smoked paprika
- 28 ounces canned tomatoes, crushed
- 1 teaspoon oregano, dried
- 1 teaspoon thyme, dried
- 1 teaspoon marjoram, dried
- A pinch of cayenne pepper
- Salt and black pepper to the taste

Directions:
1. In your Crock Pot, mix garlic with bell pepper, onion, water, okra, corn, paprika, tomatoes, oregano, thyme, marjoram, cayenne, salt and pepper, cover, cook on Low for 8 hours, divide between plates and serve as a side dish.

Nutrition Info:
- calories 182, fat 3, fiber 6, carbs 8, protein 5

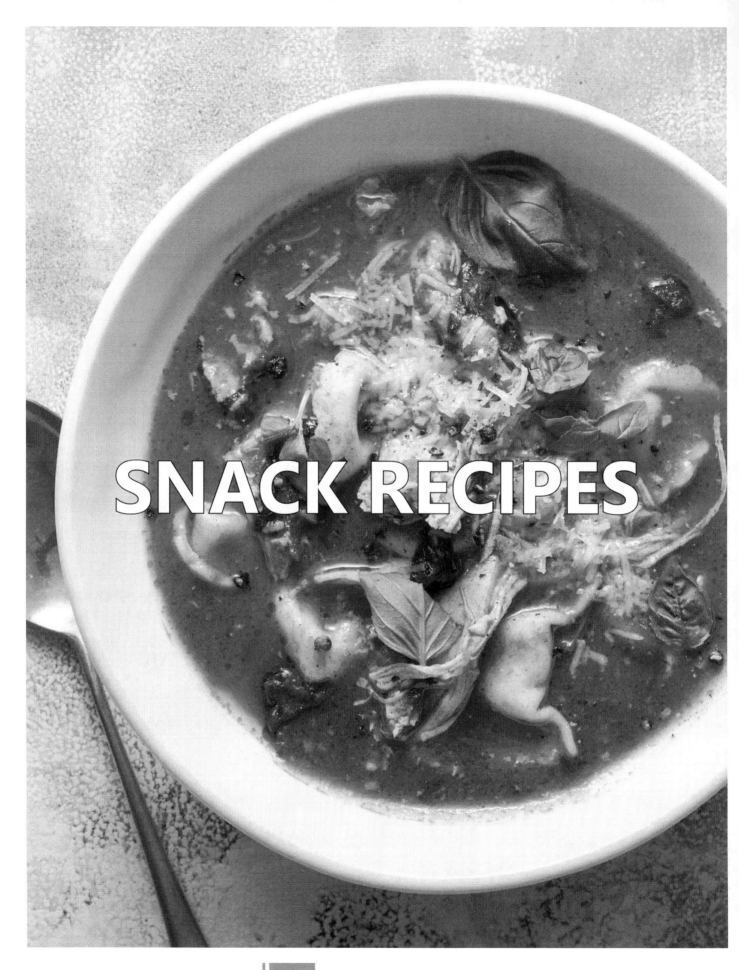

SNACK RECIPES

Bean Pesto Dip

Servings: 8
Cooking Time: 6 Hrs

Ingredients:
- 10 oz. refried beans
- 1 tbsp pesto sauce
- 1 tsp salt
- 7 oz. Cheddar cheese, shredded
- 1 tsp paprika
- 1 cup of salsa
- 4 tbsp sour cream
- 2-oz. cream cheese
- 1 tsp dried dill

Directions:
1. Mix pesto with salt, salsa, sour cream, dill, beans, cheese, paprika, and cream cheese in the Crock Pot.
2. Put the cooker's lid on and set the cooking time to 6 hours on Low settings.
3. Once Crock Pot, blend the mixture using a hand blender.
4. Serve fresh.

Nutrition Info:
- Per Serving: Calories: 102, Total Fat: 6.3g, Fiber: 1g, Total Carbs: 7.43g, Protein: 5g

Slow-cooked Lemon Peel

Servings: 80 Pieces
Cooking Time: 4 Hrs

Ingredients:
- 5 big lemons, peel cut into strips
- 2 and ¼ cups white sugar
- 5 cups of water

Directions:
1. Spread the lemon peel in the Crock Pot and top it with sugar and water.
2. Put the cooker's lid on and set the cooking time to 4 hours on Low settings.
3. Drain the cooked peel and serve.

Nutrition Info:

- Per Serving: Calories: 7, Total Fat: 1g, Fiber: 1g, Total Carbs: 2g, Protein: 1g

Zucchini Spread

Servings: 2
Cooking Time: 6 Hours

Ingredients:
- 1 tablespoon walnuts, chopped
- 2 zucchinis, grated
- 1 cup heavy cream
- 1 teaspoon balsamic vinegar
- 1 tablespoon tahini paste
- 1 tablespoon chives, chopped

Directions:
1. In your Crock Pot, combine the zucchinis with the cream, walnuts and the other ingredients, whisk, put the lid on and cook on Low for 6 hours.
2. Blend using an immersion blender, divide into bowls and serve as a party spread.

Nutrition Info:
- calories 221, fat 6, fiber 5, carbs 9, protein 3

Mixed Nuts

Servings: 6
Cooking Time: 40 Minutes

Ingredients:
- ½ tsp cooking spray
- 1 tsp chili flakes
- 1 tsp ground cinnamon
- 2 oz. butter, melted
- 1 tsp salt
- 1 cup peanuts
- 1 cup cashew
- 1 cup walnuts
- 3 tbsp maple syrup

Directions:
1. Toss cashew, peanuts, and walnuts in a baking sheet and bake for 10 minutes at 350 degrees F.
2. Toss the nuts after every 2 minutes of cooking.

3. Mix chili flakes, salt, and cinnamon ground in a bowl.
4. Transfer the nuts to the Crock Pot and drizzle spice mixture on top.
5. Whisk maple syrup and melted butter in a bowl and pour over the nuts.
6. Put the cooker's lid on and set the cooking time to 20 minutes on High settings.
7. Stir the nuts well, then continue cooking for another 20 minutes on High setting.
8. Serve.

Nutrition Info:
- Per Serving: Calories: 693, Total Fat: 55.4g, Fiber: 5g, Total Carbs: 39.16g, Protein: 20g

Candied Pecans

Servings: 4
Cooking Time: 3 Hours

Ingredients:
- 1 cup white sugar
- 1 and ½ tablespoons cinnamon powder
- ½ cup brown sugar
- 1 egg white, whisked
- 4 cups pecans
- 2 teaspoons vanilla extract
- ¼ cup water

Directions:
1. In a bowl, mix white sugar with cinnamon, brown sugar and vanilla and stir.
2. Dip pecans in egg white, then in sugar mix and put them in your Crock Pot, also add the water, cover and cook on Low for 3 hours.
3. Divide into bowls and serve as a snack.

Nutrition Info:
- calories 152, fat 4, fiber 7, carbs 16, protein 6

Bourbon Sausage Bites

Servings: 12
Cooking Time: 3 Hours And 5 Minutes

Ingredients:
- 1/3 cup bourbon
- 1 pound smoked sausage, sliced
- 12 ounces chili sauce
- ¼ cup brown sugar
- 2 tablespoons yellow onion, grated

Directions:

1. Heat up a pan over medium-high heat, add sausage slices, brown them for 2 minutes on each side, drain them on paper towels and transfer to your Crock Pot.
2. Add chili sauce, sugar, onion and bourbon, toss to coat, cover and cook on Low for 3 hours.
3. Divide into bowls and serve as a snack.

Nutrition Info:
- calories 190, fat 11, fiber 1, carbs 12, protein 5

Pineapple And Tofu Salsa

Servings: 2
Cooking Time: 6 Hours

Ingredients:
- ½ cup firm tofu, cubed
- 1 cup pineapple, peeled and cubed
- 1 cup cherry tomatoes, halved
- ½ tablespoons sesame oil
- 1 tablespoon soy sauce
- ½ cup pineapple juice
- ½ tablespoon ginger, grated
- 1 garlic clove, minced

Directions:
1. In your Crock Pot, mix the tofu with the pineapple and the other ingredients, toss, put the lid on and cook on Low for 6 hours.
2. Divide into bowls and serve as an appetizer.

Nutrition Info:
- calories 201, fat 5, fiber 7, carbs 15, protein 4

Maple Glazed Turkey Strips

Servings: 8
Cooking Time: 3.5 Hours

Ingredients:
- 15 oz. turkey fillets, cut into strips
- 2 tbsp honey
- 1 tbsp maple syrup
- 1 tsp cayenne pepper
- 1 tbsp butter
- 1 tsp paprika
- 1 tsp oregano
- 1 tsp dried dill
- 2 tbsp mayo

Directions:
1. Place the turkey strips in the Crock Pot.
2. Add all other spices, herbs, and mayo on top of the turkey.

3. Put the cooker's lid on and set the cooking time to 3 hours on High settings.
4. During this time, mix honey with maples syrup and melted butter in a bowl.
5. Pour this honey glaze over the turkey evenly.
6. Put the cooker's lid on and set the cooking time to 30 minutes on High settings.
7. Serve warm.

Nutrition Info:
- Per Serving: Calories: 295, Total Fat: 25.2g, Fiber: 0g, Total Carbs: 6.82g, Protein: 10g

Cauliflower Dip

Servings: 2
Cooking Time: 5 Hours

Ingredients:
- 1 cup cauliflower florets
- ½ cup heavy cream
- 1 tablespoon tahini paste
- ½ cup white mushrooms, chopped
- 2 garlic cloves, minced
- 2 tablespoons lemon juice
- 1 tablespoon basil, chopped
- 1 teaspoon rosemary, dried
- A pinch of salt and black pepper

Directions:
1. In your Crock Pot, mix the cauliflower with the cream, tahini paste and the other ingredients, toss, put the lid on and cook on Low for 5 hours.
2. Transfer to a blender, pulse well, divide into bowls and serve as a party dip.

Nutrition Info:
- calories 301, fat 7, fiber 6, carbs 10, protein 6

Veggie Spread

Servings: 4
Cooking Time: 7 Hours

Ingredients:
- 1 cup carrots, sliced
- 1 and ½ cups cauliflower florets
- 1/3 cup cashews
- ½ cup turnips, chopped
- 2 and ½ cups water
- 1 cup almond milk
- 1 teaspoon garlic powder
- Salt and black pepper to the taste

- ¼ teaspoon smoked paprika
- ¼ teaspoon mustard powder
- A pinch of salt

Directions:
1. In your Crock Pot, mix carrots with cauliflower, cashews, turnips and water, stir, cover and cook on Low for 7 hours.
2. Drain, transfer to a blender, add almond milk, garlic powder, paprika, mustard powder, salt and pepper, blend well, divide into bowls and serve as a snack.

Nutrition Info:
- calories 291, fat 7, fiber 4, carbs 14, protein 3

Spinach And Walnuts Dip

Servings: 2
Cooking Time: 2 Hours

Ingredients:
- ½ cup heavy cream
- ½ cup walnuts, chopped
- 1 cup baby spinach
- 1 garlic clove, chopped
- 1 tablespoon mayonnaise
- Salt and black pepper to the taste

Directions:
1. In your Crock Pot, mix the spinach with the walnuts and the other ingredients, toss, put the lid on and cook on High for 2 hours.
2. Blend using an immersion blender, divide into bowls and serve as a party dip.

Nutrition Info:
- calories 260, fat 4, fiber 2, carbs 12, protein 5

Sugary Chicken Wings

Servings: 24
Cooking Time: 6 Hours

Ingredients:
- 1 teaspoon garlic powder
- ½ cup brown sugar
- ¾ cup white sugar
- 1 teaspoon ginger powder
- 1 cup soy sauce
- ¼ cup pineapple juice
- ¾ cup water
- ¼ cup olive oil
- 24 chicken wings

Directions:

1. In a bowl, mix chicken wings with garlic powder, brown sugar, white sugar, ginger powder, soy sauce, pineapple juice, water and oil, whisk well and leave aside for 2 hours in the fridge.

2. Transfer chicken wings to your Crock Pot, add 1 cup of the marinade, cover and cook on Low for 6 hours.

3. Serve chicken wings warm.

Nutrition Info:
- calories 140, fat 7, fiber 1, carbs 12, protein 6

Nuts Bowls

Servings: 2
Cooking Time: 2 Hours

Ingredients:
- 2 tablespoons almonds, toasted
- 2 tablespoons pecans, halved and toasted
- 2 tablespoons hazelnuts, toasted and peeled
- 2 tablespoons sugar
- ½ cup coconut cream
- 2 tablespoons butter, melted
- A pinch of cinnamon powder
- A pinch of cayenne pepper

Directions:
1. In your Crock Pot, mix the nuts with the sugar and the other ingredients, toss, put the lid on, cook on Low for 2 hours, divide into bowls and serve as a snack.

Nutrition Info:
- calories 125, fat 3, fiber 2, carbs 5, protein 5

Chickpeas Salsa

Servings: 2
Cooking Time: 6 Hours

Ingredients:
- 1 cup canned chickpeas, drained
- 1 cup veggie stock
- ½ cup black olives, pitted and halved
- 1 small yellow onion, chopped
- ¼ tablespoon ginger, grated
- 4 garlic cloves, minced
- ¼ tablespoons coriander, ground
- ¼ tablespoons red chili powder
- ¼ tablespoons garam masala
- 1 tablespoon lemon juice

Directions:
1. In your Crock Pot, mix the chickpeas with the

stock, olives and the other ingredients, toss, put the lid on and cook on Low for 6 hours.

2. Divide into bowls and serve as an appetizer.

Nutrition Info:
- calories 355, fat 5, fiber 14, carbs 16, protein 11

Chickpea Hummus

Servings: 10
Cooking Time: 8 Hrs

Ingredients:
- 1 cup chickpeas, dried
- 2 tbsp olive oil
- 3 cup of water
- A pinch of salt and black pepper
- 1 garlic clove, minced
- 1 tbsp lemon juice

Directions:
1. Add chickpeas, salt, water, and black pepper to the Crock Pot.

2. Put the cooker's lid on and set the cooking time to 8 hours on Low settings.

3. Drain and transfer the chickpeas to a blender jug.

4. Add salt, black pepper, lemon juice, garlic, and olive oil.

5. Blend the chickpeas dip until smooth.

6. Serve.

Nutrition Info:
- Per Serving: Calories: 211, Total Fat: 6g, Fiber: 7g, Total Carbs: 8g, Protein: 4g

Apple Sausage Snack

Servings: 15
Cooking Time: 2 Hrs

Ingredients:
- 2 lbs. sausages, sliced
- 18 oz. apple jelly
- 9 oz. Dijon mustard

Directions:
1. Add sausage slices, apple jelly, and mustard to the Crock Pot.

2. Put the cooker's lid on and set the cooking time to 2 hours on Low settings.

3. Serve fresh.

Nutrition Info:
- Per Serving: Calories: 200, Total Fat: 3g, Fiber: 1g, Total Carbs: 9g, Protein: 10g

Potato Salsa

Servings: 6
Cooking Time: 8 Hours

Ingredients:
- 1 sweet onion, chopped
- ¼ cup white vinegar
- 2 tablespoons mustard
- Salt and black pepper to the taste
- 1 and ½ pounds gold potatoes, cut into medium cubes
- ¼ cup dill, chopped
- 1 cup celery, chopped
- Cooking spray

Directions:
1. Spray your Crock Pot with cooking spray, add onion, vinegar, mustard, salt and pepper and whisk well.
2. Add celery and potatoes, toss them well, cover and cook on Low for 8 hours.
3. Divide salad into small bowls, sprinkle dill on top and serve.

Nutrition Info:
- calories 251, fat 6, fiber 7, carbs 12, protein 7

Chicken Meatballs

Servings: 2
Cooking Time: 7 Hours

Ingredients:
- A pinch of red pepper flakes, crushed
- ½ pound chicken breast, skinless, boneless, ground
- 1 egg, whisked
- ½ cup salsa Verde
- 1 teaspoon oregano, dried
- ½ teaspoon chili powder
- ½ teaspoon rosemary, dried
- 1 tablespoon parsley, chopped
- A pinch of salt and black pepper

Directions:
1. In a bowl, mix the chicken with the egg and the other ingredients except the salsa, stir well and shape medium meatballs out of this mix.
2. Put the meatballs in the Crock Pot, add the salsa Verde, toss gently, put the lid on and cook on Low for 7 hours.
3. Arrange the meatballs on a platter and serve.

Nutrition Info:
- calories 201, fat 4, fiber 5, carbs 8, protein 2

Cauliflower Bites

Servings: 2
Cooking Time: 4 Hours

Ingredients:
- 2 cups cauliflower florets
- 1 tablespoon Italian seasoning
- 1 tablespoon sweet paprika
- 2 tablespoons tomato sauce
- 1 teaspoon sweet paprika
- 1 tablespoon olive oil
- ¼ cup veggie stock

Directions:
1. In your Crock Pot, mix the cauliflower florets with the Italian seasoning and the other ingredients, toss, put the lid on and cook on Low for 4 hours.
2. Divide into bowls and serve as a snack.

Nutrition Info:
- calories 251, fat 4, fiber 6, carbs 7, protein 3

Bacon Fingerling Potatoes

Servings: 15
Cooking Time: 8 Hours

Ingredients:
- 2 lb. fingerling potatoes
- 8 oz. bacon
- 1 tsp onion powder
- 1 tsp chili powder
- 1 tsp garlic powder
- 1 tsp paprika
- 3 tbsp butter
- 1 tsp dried dill
- 1 tbsp rosemary

Directions:
1. Grease the base of your Crock Pot with butter.
2. Spread the fingerling potatoes in the buttered cooker.
3. Mix all the spices, herbs, and bacon in a bowl.
4. Spread bacon-spice mixture over the lingering potatoes.
5. Put the cooker's lid on and set the cooking time to 8 hours on Low settings.
6. Serve warm.

Nutrition Info:
- Per Serving: Calories: 117, Total Fat: 6.9g, Fiber: 2g, Total Carbs: 12.07g, Protein: 3g

Mozzarella Basil Tomatoes

Servings: 8
Cooking Time: 30 Minutes

Ingredients:
- 3 tbsp fresh basil
- 1 tsp chili flakes
- 5 oz. Mozzarella, sliced
- 4 large tomatoes, sliced
- 1 tbsp olive oil
- 1 tsp minced garlic
- ½ tsp onion powder
- ½ tsp cilantro

Directions:
1. Whisk olive oil with onion powder, cilantro, garlic, and chili flakes in a bowl.
2. Rub all the tomato slices with this cilantro mixture.
3. Top each tomato slice with cheese slice and then place another tomato slice on top to make a sandwich.
4. Insert a toothpick into each tomato sandwich to seal it.
5. Place them in the base of the Crock Pot.
6. Put the cooker's lid on and set the cooking time to 20 minutes on High settings.
7. Garnish with basil.
8. Enjoy.

Nutrition Info:
- Per Serving: Calories: 59, Total Fat: 1.9g, Fiber: 2g, Total Carbs: 4.59g, Protein: 7g

Simple Salsa

Servings: 6
Cooking Time: 5 Hours

Ingredients:
- 7 cups tomatoes, chopped
- 1 green bell pepper, chopped
- 1 red bell pepper, chopped
- 2 yellow onions, chopped
- 4 jalapenos, chopped
- ¼ cup apple cider vinegar
- 1 teaspoon coriander, ground
- 1 tablespoon cilantro, chopped
- 3 tablespoons basil, chopped
- Salt and black pepper to the taste

Directions:
1. In your Crock Pot, mix tomatoes with green and red peppers, onions, jalapenos, vinegar, coriander, salt and pepper, stir, cover and cook on Low for 5 hours.
2. Add basil and cilantro, stir, divide into bowls and serve.

Nutrition Info:
- calories 172, fat 3, fiber 5, carbs 8, protein 4

Almond, Zucchini, Parmesan Snack

Servings: 6 (5.1 Ounces Per Serving)
Cooking Time: 1 Hour And 40 Minutes

Ingredients:
- 3 eggs, organic
- 2 zucchinis, thinly sliced
- 1 cup almonds, ground
- 1 cup Parmesan cheese, grated
- Salt and pepper to taste
- Olive oil
- 1 teaspoon oregano
- 1 cup almond flour

Directions:
1. Wash, clean, and slice the zucchini. Salt and set aside on a paper towel. On a plate, combine Parmesan cheese, almonds, oregano, salt, and pepper and set aside. On another shallow plate, spread the almond flour. In a bowl, beat eggs with salt and pepper. Start by dipping zucchini rounds in flour, dip in the eggs, then dredge in almond mixture, pressing on them to coat. Pour olive oil in Crock-Pot and add the zucchini slices; cover and cook for 1 ½ hours on HIGH. Serve hot.

Nutrition Info:
- Calories: 303.33, Total Fat: 24.22 g, Saturated Fat: 3.61 g, Cholesterol: 78.01 mg, Sodium: 160.81 mg, Potassium: 494.68 mg, Total Carbohydrates: 11.09 g, Fiber: 5.23 g, Sugar: 3.62 g, Protein: 14.65 g

Cashew Dip

Servings: 10
Cooking Time: 3 Hours

Ingredients:
- 1 cup water
- 1 cup cashews
- 10 ounces hummus
- ¼ teaspoon garlic powder
- ¼ teaspoon onion powder
- A pinch of salt and black pepper
- ¼ teaspoon mustard powder

• 1 teaspoon apple cider vinegar

Directions:

1. In your Crock Pot, mix water with cashews, salt and pepper, stir, cover and cook on High for 3 hours.
2. Transfer to your blender, add hummus, garlic powder, onion powder, mustard powder and vinegar, pulse well, divide into bowls and serve.

Nutrition Info:

• calories 192, fat 7, fiber 7, carbs 12, protein 4

Onion Dip

Servings: 2
Cooking Time: 8 Hours

Ingredients:

• 2 cups yellow onions, chopped
• A pinch of salt and black pepper
• 1 tablespoon olive oil
• ½ cup heavy cream
• 2 tablespoons mayonnaise

Directions:

1. In your Crock Pot, mix the onions with the cream and the other ingredients, whisk, put the lid on and cook on Low for 8 hours.
2. Divide into bowls and serve as a party dip.

Nutrition Info:

• calories 240, fat 4, fiber 4, carbs 9, protein 7

Beef And Chipotle Dip

Servings: 10
Cooking Time: 2 Hours

Ingredients:

• 8 ounces cream cheese, soft
• 2 tablespoons yellow onion, chopped
• 2 tablespoons mayonnaise
• 2 ounces hot pepper Monterey Jack cheese, shredded
• ¼ teaspoon garlic powder
• 2 chipotle chilies in adobo sauce, chopped
• 2 ounces dried beef, chopped
• ¼ cup pecans, chopped

Directions:

1. In your Crock Pot, mix cream cheese with onion, mayo, Monterey Jack cheese, garlic powder, chilies and dried beef, stir, cover and cook on Low for 2 hours.
2. Add pecans, stir, divide into bowls and serve.

Nutrition Info:

• calories 130, fat 11, fiber 1, carbs 3, protein 4

Crab Dip

Servings: 6
Cooking Time: 2 Hours

Ingredients:

• 12 ounces cream cheese
• ½ cup parmesan, grated
• ½ cup mayonnaise
• ½ cup green onions, chopped
• 2 garlic cloves, minced
• Juice of 1 lemon
• 1 and ½ tablespoon Worcestershire sauce
• 1 and ½ teaspoons old bay seasoning
• 12 ounces crabmeat

Directions:

1. In your Crock Pot, mix cream cheese with parmesan, mayo, green onions, garlic, lemon juice, Worcestershire sauce, old bay seasoning and crabmeat, stir, cover and cook on Low for 2 hours.
2. Divide into bowls and serve as a dip.

Nutrition Info:

• calories 200, fat 4, fiber 6, carbs 12, protein 3

Creamy Mushroom Spread

Servings: 2
Cooking Time: 4 Hours

Ingredients:

• 1 pound mushrooms, sliced
• 3 garlic cloves, minced
• 1 cup heavy cream
• 2 teaspoons smoked paprika
• Salt and black pepper to the taste
• 2 tablespoons parsley, chopped

Directions:

1. In your Crock Pot, mix the mushrooms with the garlic and the other ingredients, whisk, put the lid on and cook on Low for 4 hours.
2. Whisk, divide into bowls and serve as a party spread.

Nutrition Info:

• calories 300, fat 6, fiber 12, carbs 16, protein 6

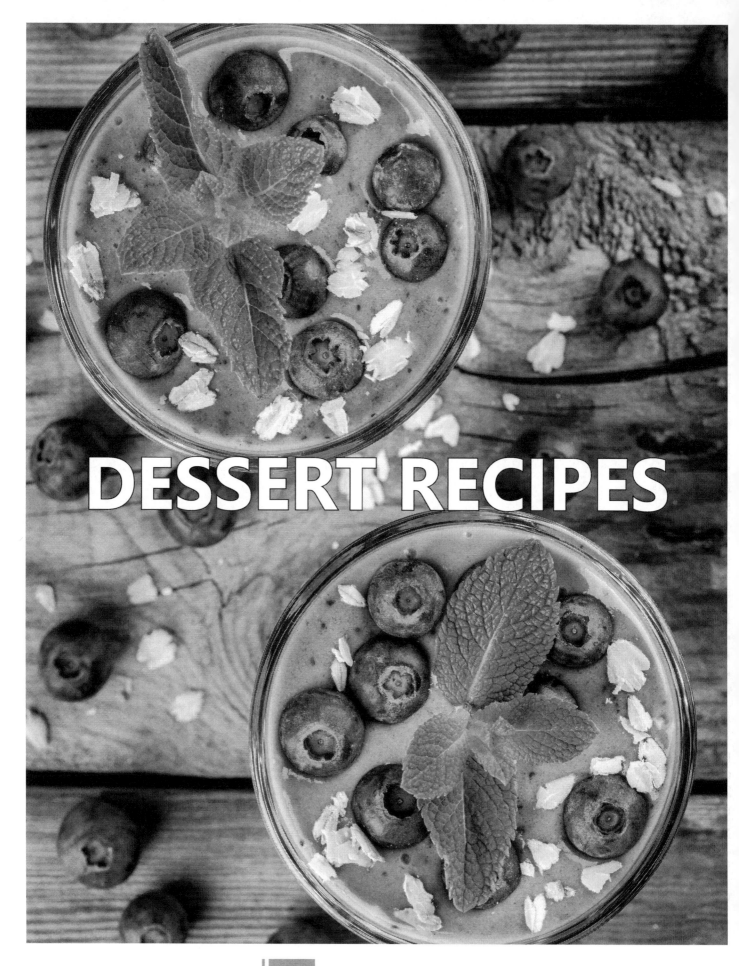

DESSERT RECIPES

Dessert Recipes

Glazed Bacon

Servings:4
Cooking Time: 2 Hours

Ingredients:
- 4 bacon slices
- 1 tablespoon butter
- 3 tablespoons water
- 5 tablespoons maple syrup

Directions:
1. Put all ingredients in the Crock Pot.
2. Close the lid and cook the dessert on High for 2 hours.
3. Then transfer the bacon in the serving plates and top with maple syrup mixture from the Crock Pot.

Nutrition Info:
- Per Serving: 193 calories, 7.1g protein, 17g carbohydrates, 10.9g fat, 0g fiber, 29mg cholesterol, 462mg sodium, 159mg potassium.

Lemon Cream

Servings: 4
Cooking Time: 1 Hour

Ingredients:
- 1 cup heavy cream
- 1 teaspoon lemon zest, grated
- ¼ cup lemon juice
- 8 ounces mascarpone cheese

Directions:
1. In your Crock Pot, mix heavy cream with mascarpone, lemon zest and lemon juice, stir, cover and cook on Low for 1 hour.
2. Divide into dessert glasses and keep in the fridge until you serve.

Nutrition Info:
- calories 165, fat 7, fiber 0, carbs 7, protein 4

Sweet Corn Ramekins

Servings:2
Cooking Time: 5 Hours

Ingredients:
- 1 cup sweet corn kernels
- ½ cup coconut cream
- 2 tablespoons condensed milk
- 1 teaspoon butter, softened

Directions:
1. Mix corn kernels with coconut cream and condensed milk.
2. Then grease the ramekins with softened butter.
3. Put the corn kernels mixture in the ramekins.
4. Transfer them in the Crock Pot and close the lid.
5. Cook the meal on Low for 5 hours.

Nutrition Info:
- Per Serving: 283 calories, 5.1g protein, 29.1g carbohydrates, 18.6g fat, 2.9g fiber, 12mg cholesterol, 291mg sodium, 340mg potassium.

Glazed Carrot With Whipped Cream

Servings:6
Cooking Time: 2.5 Hours

Ingredients:
- 1 cup whipped cream
- 3 cups baby carrot
- 4 tablespoons maple syrup
- 1 teaspoon ground cinnamon
- 1 tablespoon lemon juice
- 1 teaspoon lime zest, grated
- ½ cup of water

Directions:
1. Mix carrot with ground cinnamon, lemon juice, lime zest, and water.
2. Add maple syrup and transfer the mixture in the Crock Pot.
3. Cook the carrots on High for 2.5 hours.
4. Then cool the carrots and transfer them in the bowls.

5. Top the dessert with whipped cream.

Nutrition Info:
• Per Serving: 120 calories, 0.9g protein, 5.8g carbohydrates, 6.3g fat, 2.3g fiber, 22mg cholesterol, 64mg sodium, 220mg potassium.

Melon Pudding

Servings:3
Cooking Time: 3 Hours

Ingredients:
• 1 cup melon, chopped
• ¼ cup of coconut milk
• 2 tablespoons cornstarch
• 1 teaspoon vanilla extract

Directions:
1. Blend the melon until smooth and mix with coconut milk, cornstarch, and vanilla extract.
2. Transfer the mixture in the Crock Pot and cook the pudding on low for 3 hours.

Nutrition Info:
• Per Serving: 88 calories, 0.9g protein, 10.4g carbohydrates, 4.9g fat, 1g fiber, 0mg cholesterol, 12mg sodium, 194mg potassium.

Dump Cake

Servings:8
Cooking Time: 5 Hours

Ingredients:
• 1 cupcake mix
• 1 teaspoon vanilla extract
• ½ teaspoon ground nutmeg
• 1 tablespoon butter, melted
• 2 eggs, beaten
• 1 teaspoon lemon zest, grated
• ½ cup heavy cream
• 4 pecans, chopped

Directions:
1. In the bowl mix all ingredients except pecans.
2. The line the Crock Pot with baking paper and pour the dough inside.
3. Flatten the batter and top with pecans.
4. Close the lid and cook the dump cake for 5 hours on Low.
5. Cook the cooked cake well before serving.

Nutrition Info:
• Per Serving: 245 calories, 3.8g protein, 27g carbohy-

drates, 13.9g fat, 1.1g fiber, 55mg cholesterol, 246mg sodium, 90mg potassium

Coffee Cookies

Servings:12
Cooking Time: 4 Hours

Ingredients:
• 2 eggs, beaten
• 1 tablespoon coffee beans, grinded
• 1 teaspoon baking powder
• ½ cup butter, softened
• 2 cups flour
• ¼ cup of sugar
• 1 teaspoon sunflower oil

Directions:
1. Brush the Crock Pot bowl with sunflower oil.
2. Then mix all remaining ingredients in the mixing bowl.
3. Knead the dough and cut it into small pieces.
4. Roll the dough pieces into small balls and make the small cut in the center of every ball (to get the shape of the cocoa bean).
5. Put the cocoa beans in the Crock Pot in one layer and close the lid.
6. Cook them on High for 2 hours.
7. Repeat the same steps with remaining cookies.

Nutrition Info:
• Per Serving: 174 calories, 3.2g protein, 20.3g carbohydrates, 9g fat, 0.6g fiber, 48mg cholesterol, 66mg sodium, 77mg potassium.

Monkey Bread

Servings: 8
Cooking Time: 5 1/4 Hours

Ingredients:
• 3 cups all-purpose flour
• 4 eggs
• 1/4 cup white sugar
• 1 teaspoon vanilla extract
• 1 1/4 cups warm milk
• 1 teaspoon active dry yeast
• 3/4 cup butter, melted
• 1 cup white sugar
• 1 1/2 teaspoons cinnamon powder

Directions:
1. Mix the flour, salt, eggs, 1/4 cup white sugar, warm

milk, vanilla and active dry yeast in the bowl of your mixer and knead for 10 minutes. Allow the dough to rise for 1 hour.

2. Transfer the dough on a floured working surface and cut it into 24-30 small pieces of dough. Roll each piece of dough into a ball.

3. Mix the sugar with cinnamon powder.

4. To finish the bread, dip each ball of dough into melted butter then roll through the cinnamon sugar.

5. Grease your crock pot and place the dough balls in the pot.

6. Cook on low settings for 4 hours.

7. Allow to cool before serving.

White Chocolate Apple Cake

Servings: 8
Cooking Time: 6 1/2 Hours

Ingredients:
- 5 eggs, separated
- 3/4 cup white sugar
- 1/2 cup butter, melted
- 1/2 cup whole milk
- 1 cup all-purpose flour
- 1 teaspoon baking powder
- 1/4 teaspoon salt
- 1/2 cup white chocolate chips
- 4 tart apples, peeled, cored and sliced
- 1/2 teaspoon cinnamon powder

Directions:
1. Mix the egg yolks with half of the sugar until double in volume. Stir in the butter and milk then fold in the flour, baking powder and salt.

2. Whip the egg whites until stiff then add the remaining sugar and whip for a few minutes until glossy and stiff. Fold this meringue into the egg yolks and flour mixture then add the chocolate chips.

3. Spoon the batter in your Crock Pot and top with apple slices.

4. Sprinkle with cinnamon and cook on low settings for 6 hours.

5. Allow to cool before slicing and serving.

S'mores Baked Sweet Potatoes

Servings: 8
Cooking Time: 3 1/2 Hours

Ingredients:
- 2 large sweet potatoes, peeled and diced

- 1 teaspoon cinnamon powder
- 2 tablespoons brown sugar
- 1 1/2 cups crushed graham crackers
- 1/4 cup butter, melted
- 1 1/2 cups dark chocolate chips
- 2 cups mini marshmallows

Directions:
1. Mix the crackers and butter in a bowl. Transfer this mixture in your Crock Pot and press it well on the bottom of the pot.

2. Mix the sweet potatoes with the cinnamon and brown sugar then transfer this mix over the crackers crust.

3. Top the potatoes with chocolate chips, followed by marshmallows.

4. Cook on low settings for 3 hours.

5. Allow the dessert to cool down slightly before serving.

Swirled Peanut Butter Cake

Servings: 10
Cooking Time: 5 1/2 Hours

Ingredients:
- 3/4 cup butter, softened
- 1 cup white sugar
- 3 eggs
- 1 teaspoon vanilla extract
- 1 cup all-purpose flour
- 1 teaspoon baking powder
- 1/4 teaspoon salt
- 1/2 cup smooth peanut butter, softened

Directions:
1. Mix the butter and sugar in a bowl for 5 minutes until creamy.

2. Add the eggs, one by one and stir in the vanilla.

3. Fold in the flour, baking powder and salt and mix gently.

4. Pour half of the batter in your Crock Pot. The remaining half, mix it with the peanut butter and spoon it into the pot.

5. Bake for 5 hours on low settings.

6. Allow the cake to cool completely before serving.

Cherry Jam

Servings:4
Cooking Time: 3 Hours

Ingredients:
- 2 cups cherries, pitted
- ½ cup of sugar
- 1 tablespoon agar
- 3 tablespoons water

Directions:
1. Mix sugar with cherries and put in the Crock Pot.
2. Then mix water and agar and pour the liquid in the Crock Pot too.
3. Stir well and close the lid.
4. Cook the jam on high for 3 hours.
5. Then transfer the jam in the glass cans and store it in the fridge for up to 2 months.

Nutrition Info:
- Per Serving: 139 calories, 0.5g protein, 36.1g carbohydrates, 0g fat, 1.5g fiber, 0mg cholesterol, 0mg sodium, 3mg potassium.

Cinnamon Plum Jam

Servings:6
Cooking Time: 6 Hours

Ingredients:
- 4 cups plums, pitted, halved
- 1 tablespoon ground cinnamon
- ½ cup brown sugar
- 1 teaspoon vanilla extract

Directions:
1. Put all ingredients in the Crock Pot and gently mix.
2. Close the lid and cook it on Low for 6 hours.

Nutrition Info:
- Per Serving: 71 calories, 0.4g protein, 18.2g carbohydrates, 0.1g fat, 1.2g fiber, 0mg cholesterol, 4mg sodium, 91mg potassium.

Slow Cooked Chocolate Cream

Servings: 6
Cooking Time: 2 1/4 Hours

Ingredients:
- 1 1/2 cups dark chocolate chips
- 1 cup evaporated milk
- 1 cup heavy cream
- 1 teaspoon vanilla extract

- 2 tablespoons butter

Directions:
1. Mix all the ingredients in your Crock Pot.
2. Cover and cook on low settings for 2 hours.
3. Allow the cream to cool before using as a filling or frosting for other desserts.

Dark Chocolate Cream

Servings: 6
Cooking Time: 1 Hour

Ingredients:
- ½ cup heavy cream
- 4 ounces dark chocolate, unsweetened and chopped

Directions:
1. In your Crock Pot, mix cream with chocolate, stir, cover, cook on High for 1 hour, divide into bowls and serve cold.

Nutrition Info:
- calories 78, fat 1, fiber 1, carbs 2, protein 1

Dulce De Leche

Servings: 4
Cooking Time: 8 Hours

Ingredients:
- 1 can (14 oz.) sweetened condensed milk
- Water as needed

Directions:
1. Make 2-3 holes in the condensed milk can, preferably on the top side.
2. Place the can in your Crock Pot and add enough water to cover it 3/4.
3. Cover the crock pot with its lid and cook on low settings for 8 hours.
4. Serve the dulce de leche chilled.

Maple Chocolate Fondue

Servings: 5
Cooking Time: 4 Hrs.

Ingredients:
- 1 pinch salt
- 1 cup milk chocolate chips
- 1 cup dark chocolate chips
- ½ cup milk
- 1 tbsp butter
- ¼ tsp nutmeg

- 2 tsp maple syrup

Directions:
1. Add milk, chocolate chips, and rest of the ingredients to the insert of Crock Pot.
2. Put the cooker's lid on and set the cooking time to 4 hrs. on Low settings.
3. Serve when chilled.

Nutrition Info:
- Per Serving: Calories: 571, Total Fat: 28.7g, Fiber: 0g, Total Carbs: 74.85g, Protein: 7g

Pears With Grape Sauce

Servings: 4
Cooking Time: 1 Hr. 30 Minutes

Ingredients:
- 4 pears
- Juice and zest of 1 lemon
- 26 oz. grape juice
- 11 oz. currant jelly
- 4 garlic cloves
- ½ vanilla bean
- 4 peppercorns
- 2 rosemary springs

Directions:
1. Add grape juice, jelly, lemon juice, lemon zest, peppercorns, pears, vanilla, and rosemary in the insert of Crock Pot.
2. Put the cooker's lid on and set the cooking time to 1.5 hours on High settings.
3. Serve when chilled.

Nutrition Info:
- Per Serving: Calories: 152, Total Fat: 3g, Fiber: 5g, Total Carbs: 12g, Protein: 4g

Bread And Quinoa Pudding

Servings: 2
Cooking Time: 3 Hours

Ingredients:
- 1 cup quinoa
- 1 cup bread, cubed
- 2 cups almond milk
- 2 tablespoons honey
- 1 teaspoon cinnamon powder
- 1 teaspoon nutmeg, ground

Directions:
1. In your Crock Pot, mix the quinoa with the milk

and the other ingredients, whisk, put the lid on and cook on Low for 3 hours.
2. Divide the pudding into bowls and serve.

Nutrition Info:
- calories 981, fat 63.4, fiber 11.9, carbs 94.6, protein 19

Blueberry Dumpling Pie

Servings: 8
Cooking Time: 5 1/2 Hours

Ingredients:
- 1 1/2 pounds fresh blueberries
- 2 tablespoons cornstarch
- 1/4 cup light brown sugar
- 1 tablespoon lemon zest
- 1/2 cup butter, chilled and cubed
- 1 1/2 cups all-purpose flour
- 1/2 teaspoon salt
- 1 teaspoon baking powder
- 2 tablespoons white sugar
- 2/3 cup buttermilk, chilled

Directions:
1. Mix the blueberries, cornstarch, brown sugar and lemon zest in your Crock Pot.
2. For the dumpling topping, mix the flour, salt, baking powder, sugar and butter in a bowl and mix until sandy.
3. Stir in the buttermilk and give it a quick mix.
4. Drop spoonfuls of batter over the blueberries and cook on low settings for 5 hours.
5. Allow the dessert to cool completely before serving.

Vegan Mousse

Servings:3
Cooking Time: 2 Hours

Ingredients:
- 1 cup of coconut milk
- 2 tablespoons corn starch
- 1 teaspoon vanilla extract
- 1 avocado, pitted, pilled

Directions:
1. Mix coconut milk and corn starch until smooth and pour in the Crock Pot.
2. Add vanilla extract and cook it on High for 2 hours.
3. Then cool the mixture till room temperature and

mix with avocado.

4. Blend the mousse until fluffy and smooth.

Nutrition Info:

• Per Serving: 348 calories, 3.1g protein, 16.4g carbohydrates, 32.1g fat, 6.3g fiber, 0mg cholesterol, 16mg sodium, 537mg potassium.

Latte Vanilla Cake

Servings: 7

Cooking Time: 7 Hrs.

Ingredients:

• ½ cup pumpkin puree
• 3 cups flour
• 4 eggs
• 1 cup sugar, brown
• ½ cup of coconut milk
• 4 tbsp olive oil
• 3 tbsp espresso powder
• 2 tbsp maple syrup
• 1 tbsp vanilla extract
• 4 tbsp liquid honey
• ¼ tsp cooking spray

Directions:

1. Beat eggs with pumpkin puree, espresso powder, and brown sugar in a bowl.

2. Stir in olive oil, coconut milk, vanilla extract, liquid honey, flour, and maple syrup.

3. Whisk this pumpkin batter using a hand mixer until smooth.

4. Use cooking to grease the insert of your Crock Pot and pour the batter in it.

5. Put the cooker's lid on and set the cooking time to 7 hours on Low settings.

6. Slice and serve when chilled.

Nutrition Info:

• Per Serving: Calories: 538, Total Fat: 22g, Fiber: 2g, Total Carbs: 71.97g, Protein: 14g

Hazelnut Liqueur Cheesecake

Servings: 8

Cooking Time: 6 1/2 Hours

Ingredients:

• Crust:
• 1 cup graham crackers, crushed
• 1 cup ground hazelnuts
• 1/4 cup butter, melted

• Filling:
• 20 oz. cream cheese
• 1/2 cup hazelnut butter
• 1/4 cup hazelnut liqueur
• 1/4 cup light brown sugar
• 1/2 cup white sugar
• 4 eggs
• 1/2 cup heavy cream
• 1 pinch salt
• 1 teaspoon vanilla extract

Directions:

1. For the crust, mix the crackers, hazelnuts and butter in a bowl. Transfer the mix in your Crock Pot and press it well on the bottom of the pot.

2. For the filling, mix the cream cheese, hazelnut butter, liqueur, sugars, eggs, cream, salt and vanilla and mix well.

3. Pour the mixture over the crust and cook in the covered pot for 6 hours on low settings.

4. Serve the cheesecake chilled.

Chocolate Fudge Cake

Servings:6

Cooking Time: 2 Hours

Ingredients:

• ¼ cup of sugar
• 1 cup flour
• 1 tablespoon cocoa powder
• 1 teaspoon baking powder
• 2 oz chocolate chips
• 1/3 cup coconut milk
• 1 tablespoon coconut oil, softened

Directions:

1. Mix flour with sugar, cocoa powder, baking powder, and coconut milk.

2. Stir the mixture until smooth and place in the Crock Pot. (use the baking paper to avoid burning).

3. Then Cook the mixture on high for 2 hours.

4. Meanwhile, mix coconut oil and coconut chips and melt them in the microwave oven.

5. When the fudge is cooked, pour the chocolate chips mixture over it and leave to cool for 10-15 minutes as a minimum.

6. Cut the cake into servings.

Nutrition Info:

• Per Serving: 211 calories, 3.3g protein, 31.5g carbohydrates, 8.6g fat, 1.5g fiber, 2mg cholesterol, 11mg

sodium, 199mg potassium.

Fig Bars

Servings:6
Cooking Time: 2.5 Hours

Ingredients:
- 1 cup coconut flour
- ¼ cup of coconut oil
- 1 egg, beaten
- 1 teaspoon baking powder
- 5 oz figs, diced
- 1 teaspoon liquid honey

Directions:
1. Mix coconut flour and coconut oil and egg.
2. Add baking powder and knead the soft dough.
3. Then line the Crock Pot bottom with baking paper.
4. Put the dough inside and flatten it in the shape of the pie crust.
5. After this, mix liquid honey with diced figs and transfer them on the dough. Flatten it well.
6. Close the lid and cook the fig bars on High for 2.5 hours.

Nutrition Info:
- Per Serving: 232 calories, 4.4g protein, 29.8g carbohydrates, 12g fat, 10.3g fiber, 27mg cholesterol, 13mg sodium, 255mg potassium.

Spiced Raisins Tapioca Pudding

Servings: 6
Cooking Time: 6 1/4 Hours

Ingredients:
- 1 cup tapioca pearls
- 3 cups whole milk
- 1 cup golden raisins
- 1 cinnamon stick
- 1 star anise
- 2 whole cloves
- 1/4 cup maple syrup

Directions:
1. Combine all the ingredients in your Crock Pot.
2. Cover the pot and cook on low settings for 6 hours.
3. Allow the pudding to cool in the pot before serving.

Banana Chia Seeds Pudding

Servings:2
Cooking Time: 5 Hours

Ingredients:
- 1 cup milk
- 4 tablespoons chia seeds
- 2 bananas, chopped

Directions:
1. Mix milk with chia seeds and pour in the Crock Pot.
2. Cook the liquid on Low for 5 hours.
3. Meanwhile, put the chopped bananas in the bottom of glass jars.
4. When the pudding is cooked, pour it over the bananas.

Nutrition Info:
- Per Serving: 304 calories, 10g protein, 44.9g carbohydrates, 11.6g fat, 12.8g fiber, 10mg cholesterol, 63mg sodium, 608mg potassium.

Cumin Cookies

Servings:8
Cooking Time: 3 Hours

Ingredients:
- 1 teaspoon cumin seeds
- 1 tablespoon water
- 1 egg, beaten
- ½ cup cream cheese
- 2 cups flour
- ¼ cup of sugar
- 1 teaspoon baking powder
- ¼ cup milk
- Cooking spray

Directions:
1. Mix egg with cream cheese, flour, sugar, baking powder, and milk.
2. Knead the non-sticky dough and cut it into pieces.
3. Make balls.
4. Brush every ball with water and sprinkle with cumin seeds.
5. Line the Crock Pot bowl with baking paper.
6. Put the cumin cookies inside and close the lid.
7. Cook them on High for 3 hours.

Nutrition Info:
- Per Serving: 201 calories, 5.3g protein, 31.3g carbohydrates, 6.1g fat, 0.9g fiber, 37mg cholesterol, 56mg sodium, 131mg potassium.

Recipe

....

From the kicthen of ....

Serves .... Prep time .... Cook time ....

☐ Difficulty   ☐ Easy   ☐ Medium   ☐ Hard

Ingredient

....

....

....

....

....

Directions ....

....

....

....

....

....

....

Date: _____

MY SHOPPING LIST

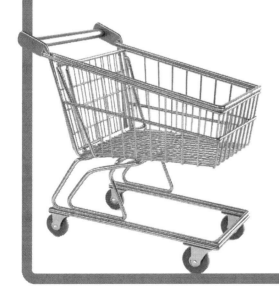

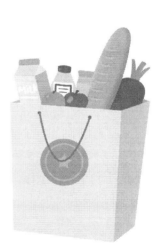

APPENDIX A: Measurement Conversions

BASIC KITCHEN CONVERSIONS & EQUIVALENTS

DRY MEASUREMENTS CONVERSION CHART

3 TEASPOONS = 1 TABLESPOON = 1/16 CUP

6 TEASPOONS = 2 TABLESPOONS = 1/8 CUP

12 TEASPOONS = 4 TABLESPOONS = 1/4 CUP

24 TEASPOONS = 8 TABLESPOONS = 1/2 CUP

36 TEASPOONS = 12 TABLESPOONS = 3/4 CUP

48 TEASPOONS = 16 TABLESPOONS = 1 CUP

METRIC TO US COOKING CONVERSIONS

OVEN TEMPERATURES

120 °C = 250 °F

160 °C = 320 °F

180° C = 350 °F

205 °C = 400 °F

220 °C = 425 °F

LIQUID MEASUREMENTS CONVERSION CHART

8 FLUID OUNCES = 1 CUP = 1/2 PINT = 1/4 QUART

16 FLUID OUNCES = 2 CUPS = 1 PINT = 1/2 QUART

32 FLUID OUNCES = 4 CUPS = 2 PINTS = 1 QUART

 = 1/4 GALLON

128 FLUID OUNCES = 16 CUPS = 8 PINTS = 4 QUARTS = 1 GALLON

BAKING IN GRAMS

1 CUP FLOUR = 140 GRAMS

1 CUP SUGAR = 150 GRAMS

1 CUP POWDERED SUGAR = 160 GRAMS

1 CUP HEAVY CREAM = 235 GRAMS

VOLUME

1 MILLILITER = 1/5 TEASPOON

5 ML = 1 TEASPOON

15 ML = 1 TABLESPOON

240 ML = 1 CUP OR 8 FLUID OUNCES

1 LITER = 34 FL. OUNCES

US TO METRIC COOKING CONVERSIONS

1/5 TSP = 1 ML

1 TSP = 5 ML

1 TBSP = 15 ML

1 FL OUNCE = 30 ML

1 CUP = 237 ML

1 PINT (2 CUPS) = 473 ML

1 QUART (4 CUPS) = .95 LITER

1 GALLON (16 CUPS) = 3.8 LITERS

1 OZ = 28 GRAMS

1 POUND = 454 GRAMS

BUTTER

1 CUP BUTTER = 2 STICKS = 8 OUNCES = 230 GRAMS = 8 TABLESPOONS

WHAT DOES 1 CUP EQUAL

1 CUP = 8 FLUID OUNCES

1 CUP = 16 TABLESPOONS

1 CUP = 48 TEASPOONS

1 CUP = 1/2 PINT

1 CUP = 1/4 QUART

1 CUP = 1/16 GALLON

1 CUP = 240 ML

WEIGHT

1 GRAM = .035 OUNCES

100 GRAMS = 3.5 OUNCES

500 GRAMS = 1.1 POUNDS

1 KILOGRAM = 35 OUNCES

BAKING PAN CONVERSIONS

1 CUP ALL-PURPOSE FLOUR = 4.5 OZ

1 CUP ROLLED OATS = 3 OZ 1 LARGE EGG = 1.7 OZ

1 CUP BUTTER = 8 OZ 1 CUP MILK = 8 OZ

1 CUP HEAVY CREAM = 8.4 OZ

1 CUP GRANULATED SUGAR = 7.1 OZ

1 CUP PACKED BROWN SUGAR = 7.75 OZ

1 CUP VEGETABLE OIL = 7.7 OZ

1 CUP UNSIFTED POWDERED SUGAR = 4.4 OZ

BAKING PAN CONVERSIONS

9-INCH ROUND CAKE PAN = 12 CUPS

10-INCH TUBE PAN =16 CUPS

11-INCH BUNDT PAN = 12 CUPS

9-INCH SPRINGFORM PAN = 10 CUPS

9 X 5 INCH LOAF PAN = 8 CUPS

9-INCH SQUARE PAN = 8 CUPS

Appendix B : Recipes Index

Made in United States
Troutdale, OR
10/27/2024

24178982R00064